# Physical Therapy
## Documentation
### From Examination to Outcome

Mia Erickson, EdD, PT, CHT, ATC
West Virginia University
Department of Human Performance and Applied Exercise Science
Morgantown, WV

Rebecca McKnight, PT, MS
Physical Therapist Assistant Program
Ozarks Technical Community College
Springfield, MO

Ralph Utzman, PhD, MPH, PT
West Virginia University
Department of Human Performance and Applied Exercise Science
Morgantown, WV

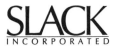

SLACK
INCORPORATED

*Delivering the best in health care information and education worldwide*

**www.slackbooks.com**

ISBN: 978-1-55642-782-4

*Physical Therapy Documentation: From Examination to Outcome Instructor's Manual* is also available from SLACK Incorporated. Don't miss this important companion to *Physical Therapy Documentation: From Examination to Outcome*. To obtain the Instructor's Manual, please visit http://www.efacultylounge.com

The procedures and practices described in this book should be implemented in a manner consistent with the professional standards set for the circumstances that apply in each specific situation. Every effort has been made to confirm the accuracy of the information presented and to correctly relate generally accepted practices. The authors, editor, and publisher cannot accept responsibility for errors or exclusions or for the outcome of the material presented herein. There is no expressed or implied warranty of this book or information imparted by it. Care has been taken to ensure that drug selection and dosages are in accordance with currently accepted/recommended practice. Due to continuing research, changes in government policy and regulations, and various effects of drug reactions and interactions, it is recommended that the reader carefully review all materials and literature provided for each drug, especially those that are new or not frequently used. Any review or mention of specific companies or products is not intended as an endorsement by the author or publisher.

SLACK Incorporated uses a review process to evaluate submitted material. Prior to publication, educators or clinicians provide important feedback on the content that we publish. We welcome feedback on this work.

Published by:     SLACK Incorporated
                  6900 Grove Road
                  Thorofare, NJ 08086 USA
                  Telephone: 856-848-1000
                  Fax: 856-848-6091
                  www.slackbooks.com

Contact SLACK Incorporated for more information about other books in this field or about the availability of our books from distributors outside the United States.

Library of Congress Cataloging-in-Publication Data

Erickson, Mia L.
 Physical therapy documentation : from examination to outcome / Mia Erickson, Rebecca McKnight, Ralph Utzman.
     p. ; cm.
 Includes bibliographical references and index.
 ISBN-13: 978-1-55642-782-4 (alk. paper)
 ISBN-10: 1-55642-782-4 (alk. paper)
 1.  Physical therapy--Documentation. 2.  Medical records. I. McKnight, Rebecca, 1969- II. Utzman, Ralph, 1966- III. Title.
 [DNLM: 1.  Medical Records. 2.  Physical Therapy (Specialty)--organization & administration. 3.  Forms and Records Control.  WB 460 E68p 2008]
 RM705.E742 2008
 615.8'2--dc22
                                                                          2008001794

Printed in the United States of America.

Last digit is print number: 10  9  8  7  6  5  4  3  2

# Physical Therapy

## Documentation

### From Examination to Outcome

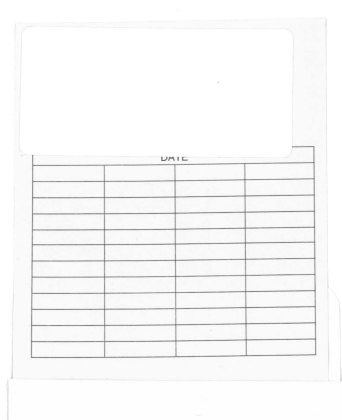

# Contents

*Physical Therapy Documentation: From Examination to Outcome Instructor's Manual* is also available from SLACK Incorporated. Don't miss this important companion to *Physical Therapy Documentation: From Examination to Outcome*. To obtain the Instructor's Manual, please visit http://www.efacultylounge.com

# Acknowledgments

I want to express my most sincere thanks and gratitude to both Becky and Ralph for working with me on this project. I never could have completed it without you. Your expertise and contributions were invaluable. Also, I would like to give a special thanks to the fabulous team of individuals at SLACK Incorporated for their patience, perseverance, dedication, and contributions throughout this process. Thank you to Jeff and Nathan, I could have never completed this without your unconditional love, support, and play dates. Finally, I thank God for placing in my life all the talented individuals who contributed to this project and for abundantly blessing me beyond what I deserve.

**Mia Erickson, EdD, PT, CHT, ATC**

I would first like to thank Mia for allowing me the opportunity to work with her on this project and I thank her and Ralph for their patience. Most importantly, I would like to acknowledge my husband and his constant support of me in my various activities. I would also like to thank my kids (Brett, Brantley, Crystal, Alicea, Bren, and Jessica) for putting up with an over committed mother/step-mother. To my Mom, thanks for the continued support of my pursuits; without her willingness to help with the kids I would not have the time or energy for anything, much less writing a book. Finally, I would like to thank my colleagues and administration at Ozarks Technical Community College for providing the flexibility in my work obligations to participate in this type of activity.

**Rebecca McKnight, PT, MS**

First, I would like to thank Mia and Becky for inviting me to participate in this wonderful project. It has been a joy to work with and learn from you both. I would also like to thank Jane Pertko, PT, GCS, who taught my first documentation class in physical therapy school. She taught the importance of documenting the PT thought process in a clear, complete, and concise way, which is more important now than ever. Finally, I would like to thank my wife, Donna, and our kids (Ryan, Nathan, Logan, and Gretchan) for their love and support.

**Ralph Utzman, PhD, MPH, PT**

# About the Authors

*Mia Erickson, EdD, PT, CHT, ATC* is currently an Associate Professor and Co-Academic Coordinator of Clinical Education at West Virginia University. She has a Bachelor's degree in Secondary Education and Athletic Training from West Virginia University. She received a Master of Science degree in Physical Therapy from the University of Indianapolis in 1996 and completed her Doctoral degree in Education at West Virginia University in 2002. She participates in clinical practice in Fairmont, WV in outpatient hand and upper extremity rehabilitation.

*Rebecca McKnight, PT, MS* is currently the Program Coordinator of the Physical Therapist Assistant Program at Ozarks Technical Community College in Springfield, MO. She also is an adjunct instructor at the Physical Therapist Program at Missouri State University. Rebecca received her Bachelor's of Science degree in Physical Therapy from St. Louis University in 1992 and her post-professional Master's of Science degree from Rocky Mountain University of Health Professions in 1999. Rebecca has recently begun a consulting business with her husband (Reach Consulting) and provides consultation related to curriculum design, development, and assessment. Rebecca is an active member of the American Physical Therapy Association, primarily within the Education Section.

*Ralph R. Utzman, PT, MPH, PhD* is Associate Professor and Co-Academic Coordinator of Clinical Education in the Division of Physical Therapy at the West Virginia University School of Medicine. He holds a Bachelor's degree in Physical Therapy and a Master's degree in Public Health from West Virginia University, and a Doctor of Philosophy degree in Health Related Sciences, Physical Therapy Track from the MCV Campus of Virginia Commonwealth University. He currently practices as part of an interdisciplinary care team for people with Parkinson's disease. He teaches in the areas of professional practice roles, practice administration, and clinical skills.

# Introduction

Thank you for choosing *Physical Therapy Documentation: From Examination to Outcome*. We believe that this book will offer you—whether you are a student, clinician, or instructor—relevant, up-to-date information for surviving the documentation maze. It is our goal for PTs to understand the importance of the day-to-day note-writing tasks while being efficient and effective.

You will notice several themes recurring throughout the text. First, we wanted to emphasize the need for showing how information is related. For example, we believe that interim, or daily notes should correspond with the initial examination and evaluative documentation. We also believe it is also important for PTs to relate information found in the subjective and objective aspects of each note with the assessment and plan portions.

Another theme that we use throughout the text is disablement. Whether you use Nagi's Framework or the ICF, the text emphasizes identifying impairments, functional deficits, and participation restriction, as well as the importance of describing how these are interrelated and how one influences another. In keeping with the disablement discussion, we believe that all physical therapy records should overtly express how interventions are influencing all aspects of disablement, including impairments and function. We also emphasize the importance of relating changes in objective data to changes in functional status.

Chapter 1 can be used in any course outlining the different disablement models and the need for a disablement framework in physical therapy. Chapters 2 through 5 can be used sequentially in an introductory course to set up basic rules for documenting. Chapter 5 is designed to provide the reader with both general and specific guidelines for documenting patient care. Chapters 6 through 9 provide practice for writing different aspects of the notes. Chapters 10 through 12 can be used to give an introduction to topics that are increasingly important in physical therapy: outcomes, reimbursement, and legal and ethical issues.

While we realize the importance and need for a variety of documentation formats, it is our experience that the SOAP format is most commonly used. However, we recognize some of the problems with it, which can be found in Chapter 4. So we decided to use the basic SOAP structure as a guide for note writing, but emphasize the importance of integrating function and showing relationships between each piece of the note.

Thank you again choosing our book. Enjoy!

## Chapter 1

# Overview of Disablement

*Mia Erickson, PT, EdD, CHT, ATC*

## Chapter Objectives

Upon completion of this chapter, the reader will be able to:

1. Discuss the need for standard disablement concepts in patient care, health policy, and research.
2. Identify events that influenced changes in disability-related terminology over the last 50 years.
3. Compare and contrast historical and contemporary disablement models.
4. Differentiate between pathology, impairment, functional limitation, disability, activity limitation, participation restrictions, and societal limitation.
5. Differentiate between the "Functioning and Disability" and "Contextual Factors" components of the ICF.
6. Describe patient examination under the ICF.
7. Examine the purpose and structure of the WHO-FIC.
8. Examine the integration of disablement in physical therapy.
9. List examples of how disablement concepts can be integrated into documentation.

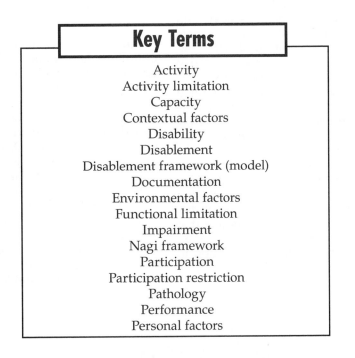

### Key Terms

Activity
Activity limitation
Capacity
Contextual factors
Disability
Disablement
Disablement framework (model)
Documentation
Environmental factors
Functional limitation
Impairment
Nagi framework
Participation
Participation restriction
Pathology
Performance
Personal factors

---

## Key Abbreviations

ADL
ICD-9
ICD-10
ICF
ICHI
ICIDH
NCMRR
WHO
WHO-FIC

---

## Introduction

One approach to defining a person's state of health comes from the biomedical model where health means free from disease.[1] An individual experiencing any departure from this normal state of physical or mental well-being is considered to have a "health condition."[2] However, the definition of health or health condition goes beyond the mere presence or absence of disease. The World Health Organization (WHO) defined health as "a state of complete physical, mental, and social well-being and not merely the absence of disease or infirmity."[3] This is sometimes referred to as the *biopsychosocial model*.

Treating and curing the health condition (or disease) is often a primary focus of health care in the biomedical model. Additionally, in traditional medical models, there is often little emphasis on how the disease or health condition affects the individual's ability to participate in society. Nevertheless, a 2004 document from the WHO put forth that a person's "health, or state of health, can only be defined in terms of an individual and that person's goals and expectations."[4(p8)] Therefore, health care providers must consider the consequences of any health condition, whether physical, mental, or emotional, that affects an individual's ability to function in society. The consequence(s) of health condition(s) affecting a person's ability to participate in society has become known as *disablement*. In essence, disablement is the gap between an individual's capabilities and the environmental or societal demands.[5]

Blending health, function, and society is not a new concept. In fact, throughout the last five decades, authors have iterated the need for inclusion of both social and cultural variables in the definition of disability. As early as 1959, Sokolow et al[6] indicated that disability should be determined on the basis of social, psychological, and vocational factors, in addition to medical factors.

## The Evolution of Disablement

Since the 1950s, the relationship between disease presence, function, and societal demands (or disablement) has been a growing area of interest, yet there has traditionally been a lack of standardized terminology for defining disablement and disablement concepts. Townsend[7] provided five different definitions that existed for the term "disability" in the 1960s, including:

1. An anatomical, physiological, or psychological abnormality

2. A chronic clinical condition altering or interrupting normal physiological or psychological processes

3. A functional limitation of ordinary activity

4. A pattern of behavior of a socially deviant kind

5. A socially defined position or status, usually of inferiority

Additionally, evaluation of disability is complex, and there has traditionally been a lack of standard evaluation tools for determining an individual's degree of disability. Early evaluation procedures included global function assessments that provide an "overall functional profile" and activity of daily living (ADL) assessments such as the Katz Index of ADL and the Barthel Index. Disease- or condition-specific instruments such as the Jebson Test of Hand Function have also been used.[8] Many more of these assessment tools (global, ADL, and disease-specific) are available today and will be discussed in subsequent chapters.

Moreover, organizations collecting disability-related data from the public have used a variety of terms and measures in their evaluation procedures. Using patient self-report, the National Center for Health Statistics asked the individual if he or she was:

1) limited, but not in a major activity; 2) limited in amount and/or type of a major activity; or 3) unable to carry out a major activity. The International Center for the Disabled and the National Council on Handicapped performed interviews with individuals who met any of the following three criteria to estimate the prevalence of disability in America: 1) inability to fully participate in work, school, or other activities; 2) having a physical disability, a seeing, hearing, or speaking impairment, an emotional or mental disability, or a learning disorder; or 3) having a perception or belief that he or she was disabled, or that others would consider him or her to be disabled.[9]

Poor standardization of terms and evaluation tools was compounded by difficulty correlating presence of disease to functional status. These problems with disablement-related terminology and evaluation were further illuminated as government agencies began providing monetary compensation to individuals with disabilities, especially when the agency was determining the amount a patient was to be awarded.[10] For example, the presence of a disease or illness does not directly translate into inability to perform self-care skills, function in the home environment, attain gainful employment, or participate in community or social activities. More often than not, it is the severity of the illness and the disease consequences that most influence the individual's functional capacity and thus determine the degree of disability (see Examples 1 and 2).

After reviewing these cases, it should be apparent that presence of disease alone should not be the sole basis for determining a patient's functional capacity or degree of disability.

Advances in medical care are prolonging the lives of individuals who once may not have survived a chronic disease or severe injury. However, increased survival does not equate to quality of life. Many individuals surviving life-threatening illnesses have long-term functional loss and disabilities. The increasing prevalence of individuals receiving disability benefits combined with poorly standardized terms and evaluation procedures that continue to exist have had a significant financial impact on society and agencies providing disability benefits.[10]

## Disablement Frameworks

The economic impact of disabilities has led US and international organizations to examine terminology, evaluation procedures, and the relationship between disease presence and functional capacity. In an effort to improve consistency, frameworks for disablement concepts have been developed to "organize information about the consequences of disease."[9(p5)] A conceptual framework is a model or guide for terminology and measurements.[5] Disablement frameworks that have emerged include: 1) *The International Classification of Functioning, Disability, and Health*, or ICF, developed by the WHO; 2) the Nagi framework, developed by Saad Nagi; and 3) the National Center for Medical Rehabilitation Research (NCMRR) disability classification scheme.

*Disablement Frameworks*

- International Classification of Functioning, Disability, and Health (ICF)
- Nagi Framework
- National Center for Medical Rehabilitation Research (NCMRR) disability classification scheme

## International Classification of Functioning, Disability, and Health

The ICF, originally known as the *International Classification of Impairments, Disabilities, and Handicaps*

(ICIDH), was endorsed by the 54th World Health Assembly and released in 2001. The operational definitions listed below have been endorsed by the WHO as part of the ICF[11(pp3,12-14)]:

- *Activity*: Completion of a task or action by an individual
- *Participation*: Involvement in a life situation
- *Impairment*: A problem with body function (physiological or psychological) or structure (limb, organ) such as a deviation from what would be considered normal. Impairments may be directly related to the health condition or a result of another impairment (eg, postural abnormalities due to muscle imbalance). Impairments can be considered permanent or temporary; progressive, regressive, or static; intermittent or continuous; slight or severe; fluctuating
- *Activity limitations*: Difficulties that might be encountered by an individual who is attempting to complete a task or carry out an activity
- *Participation restrictions*: Problems an individual might face while involved in life situations
- *Functioning*: Encompasses bodily functions, activities, and participation
- *Disability*: Encompasses impairments, activity limitations, and participation restrictions

One aim of the ICF is to provide a common language for classifying functional status and disability according to health and health-related states.[11] In other words, the ICF blends anatomical and physiological impairments with physical function and contextual factors to describe what the individual can and cannot do. The ICF describes a person's health as it relates to the body structures, the individual's life roles and tasks, and his or her participation within society. This is accomplished by categorizing information about an individual's health condition into two distinct, but related parts: (1) Functioning and Disability and (2) Contextual Factors.[11] Each part is further divided into components, domains, constructs, positive aspects, and negative aspects (Table 1-1). Part 1, Functioning and Disability, is divided into two components, a) Body Functions and Structures and b) Activities and Participation. Part 2, Contextual Factors is comprised of both a) environmental factors and b) personal factors.

## The ICF Evaluation Scheme

Under the Body Functions and Structures component of the model, the ICF evaluation scheme provides categories of bodily (physiological) functions and anatomical or body structures to be examined (Table 1-2). These physiological and anatomical functions and structures are examined to determine if deviations

*Context*: The interrelated conditions in which something exists or occurs, ie, the environment or setting.

From: Merriam-Webster's Online Dictionary. www.m-w.com/dictionary. Accessed February 9, 2007.

from "normal" exist. This allows identification of systems that are uninvolved, or intact (positive aspects) and involved, or impaired (negative aspects).[12,13] In scoring this component, the extent of the change, or deviation from normal, is scored "0" (no impairment) through "4" (complete impairment). It may also be scored "8" (not specified) or "9" (not applicable). The nature of the impairment, or deviation from normal (scored for Body Structure only), is then scored using one of the categories listed in Table 1-2.[13]

For the next component, Activities and Participation, activities are defined as "the execution of tasks or actions," or isolated tasks or functional activities. Participation is defined as "involvement in life situations,"[13(p4)] or performance of social skills like work or community involvement. Under the Activities and Participation Component, the ICF provides a set of functional skills (Table 1-3) that are scored based on an individual's performance and capacity.[12,13] Performance, or "Extent of Participation Restrictions," is the individual's "actual performance in his or her current environment."[13(p4)] It is scored according to the amount of difficulty the individual experiences in doing things, assuming they want to do them (0=no difficulty to 4=complete difficulty, 8=not specified, or 9=not applicable).[13]

Capacity, or "Extent of Activity Limitations," is described as "direct manifestations of the health state, performed without the assistance."[13(p4)] The individual's functional capacity is scored relative to what would be normally expected, or what was normal prior to acquiring the health condition. Like performance, capacity is scored using a scale of "0" (no difficulty) through "4" (complete difficulty), or it may be scored "8" (not specified), or "9" (not applicable).[13] Using this scoring system for the Activities and Participation Component, the examiner identifies skills the individual can do (positive aspects of the health condition) as well as skills the individual is unable to do (negative aspects).

Contextual factors, including both the environmental/social setting in which the individual is functioning and personal factors or characteristics, are considered when evaluating performance (see Table 1-3).[13] Environmental factors are external factors, either immediate or global, that affect the individual as he or she interacts with society. More specifically, they "make up the physical, social, and attitudinal environment in which people conduct their lives."[13(p7)] Things that facilitate interaction with the environment (eg, wheelchair ramps) are considered "positive aspects," whereas "negative aspects" are things that prevent the individual from interacting in the environment. Examples include others' opinions or attitudes, as well

Table 1-1

# The International Classification of Functioning, Disability, and Health (ICF) *from the World Health Organization*

| | Part 1: Functioning and Disability | | Part 2: Contextual Factors | |
|---|---|---|---|---|
| Components | Body Functions and Structures | Activities and Participation | Environmental Factors | Personal Factors |
| Domains | Body functions Body structures | Life areas (tasks, actions) | External influences on functioning and disability | Internal influences on functioning and disability |
| Constructs | Change in body functions (physiological) Change in body structures (anatomical) | Capacity—Executing tasks in a standard environment Performance—Executing tasks in the current environment | Facilitating or hindering impact of features (attributes) of the physical, social, and attitudinal world | Impact of attributes of the person |
| Positive aspect | Functional and structural integrity | Activities Participation | Facilitators | Not applicable |
| | Functioning | | | |
| Negative aspect | Impairment | Activity limitation Participation restriction | Barriers/hindrances | Not applicable |
| | Disability | | | |

Reprinted with permission from the World Health Organization (WHO).

as physical barriers like curbs and stairs. Personal factors are factors that are unique to the individual, such as age, race, gender, co-morbidities, fitness level, or personal attributes. Specific positive and negative personal attributes are not listed in the framework,[11] but a space for writing individual characteristics influencing function is provided for the examiner.[13] This proposed evaluation scheme is sophisticated and complex and has taken years to develop. Okochi et al[14] performed a reliability study that indicated relatively low reliability initially that increased with evaluator experience, thus suggesting the need for proper training and education in using the instrument as a disability evaluation.

According to the WHO,[11] there is difficulty differentiating between Activities and Participation. In looking back to the proposed definitions, an activity is simply a task or action carried out by an individual, whereas participation is involvement in a life situation. The WHO has suggested ways that health care practitioners and facilities using the ICF can operationally define or differentiate between activities and participation. These include: 1) to designate some functional skills as activities and some as participation (no overlap), 2) to designate some functional skills as

activities and some as participation (with overlap), 3) to name detailed skills as activities and broad skills as participation, or 4) to call all skills "activities and participation," not differentiating between the two.[11]

Jette et al[15] indicated that "differentiation is essential if the ICF is to achieve acceptance by individuals, organizations, and associations as an international classification of human functioning and disability."(p145) These investigators tested the hypothesis that distinct activities and participation could be identified using a patient self-report questionnaire (The Late Life Function and Disability Instrument). They reported that for this group of subjects, Activities and Participation were distinct categories with mobility and daily activities in the Activity dimension and social participation activities in the Participation dimension.[15] More recently, using subjects status post-distal radius fracture, Harris et al[16] indicated that the ICF framework was useful in categorizing the health effects of radius fracture and patient self-reported questionnaires should provide insight to impairments, activity limitation, and participation restrictions for these patients.

The ICF is one classification system under the World Health Organization Family of International

Table 1-2

## Categories and Scoring for "Body Functions and Structures" Using the ICF

| Categories of "Body Functions" | Extent of Change[a] | Nature of Change[b] |
|---|---|---|
| 1. Mental<br>2. Sensory and Pain<br>3. Voice and Speech<br>4. Cardiovascular, Hematological, Immunological, and Respiratory<br>5. Digestive, Metabolic, and Endocrine<br>6. Genitourinary and Reproductive<br>7. Neuromuscular and Movement-Related Disorders<br>8. Skin and related structures | | Not scored under "Function" |
| Categories of "Body Structures" | Extent of Change[a] | Nature of Change[b] |
| 1. Nervous System<br>2. Eye, Ear and other related structures<br>3. Structures related to Voice and Speech<br>4. Structures of/related to the Cardiovascular, Hematological, Immunological, and Respiratory Systems<br>5. Structures of/related to the Digestive, Metabolic, and Endocrine Systems<br>6. Structures of/related to the Genitourinary and Reproductive Systems<br>7. Structures related to Movement<br>8. Structures of/related to the Skin | | |

Scoring

[a] "0" (no impairment) through "4" (complete impairment), or it may be scored "8" (not specified) or "9" (not applicable)

[b] 0: No change in structure
 1: Total absence
 2: Partial absence
 3: Additional part
 4: Aberrant dimensions
 5: Discontinuity
 6: Deviating position
 7: Qualitative change in body structure, including fluid accumulation
 8: Not specified
 9: Not applicable

From World Health Organization. ICF Checklist. 2003. Available at: http://www3.who.int/icf/checklist/icf-checklist.pdf. Accessed February 1, 2006.

Classifications, or WHO-FIC. The primary purpose of the WHO-FIC is to provide a uniform, standard language to describe disease, health, disability, function, and interventions. Other WHO-FIC classification systems are the *International Statistical Classification of Diseases and Related Health Problems, Tenth Revision* (ICD-10), a classification system for medical diagnoses and diseases, and the *International Classification of* *Health Interventions* (ICHI), a classification of curative and preventative health interventions.[17] The three classifications (ICF, ICD-10, and ICHI) are designed to complement one another. The ICHI is still in testing phases,[17] but the WHO recommends that the ICD-10 and ICF be used together as frameworks for classifying disease along with its associated function and disability.[11] Currently, the US health care

Table 1-3

## List of Functional Skills and Scoring for the Activities and Participation Component of the ICF

### Activities and Participation

| Functional Skill | Performance[a,e] | | | Capacity[d,e] |
|---|---|---|---|---|
| | Overall score[e] | Environmental Factors[b] | Personal Factors[c] | |
| 1. Learning and applying knowledge | | | | |
| 2. General tasks and demands | | | | |
| 3. Communication | | | | |
| 4. Mobility | | | | |
| 5. Self-care | | | | |
| 6. Domestic life | | | | |
| 7. Interpersonal interactions and relationships | | | | |
| 8. Major life areas | | | | |
| 9. Community, social, and civic life | | | | |

[a] Extent of the Participation Restrictions (Life Situations—actual performance in his or her current environment)

[b] Environmental factors allowing increased participation
  a. Products and technology
  b. Natural environment and human-made changes to the natural environment
  c. Support and relationships
  d. Attitudes
  e. Services, systems, and policies

[c] Personal characteristics unique to the individual, such as age, race, gender, co-morbidities, fitness level, or personal attributes

[d] Extent of Activity Limitations (Specific Tasks)-direct manifestation of health condition, includes activity performance; performed without assistance

[e] Scoring for Performance and Capacity: "0" (No difficulty) through "4" (Complete difficulty), or it may be scored "8" (Not specified), or "9" (Not applicable).

From World Health Organization. ICF Checklist. 2003. Available at: http://www3.who.int/icf/checklist/icf-checklist.pdf.

system uses a prior version of the ICD, the ICD-9. The WHO-FIC is recommended for use by and provided to governments, health care providers, consumers, and researchers throughout the world.[4] Standard classification systems and language facilitates storage, retrieval and comparison of disease-related data in health care systems throughout the world.[4]

## The Nagi Disablement Framework

The Nagi Disablement Framework was developed in the 1960s by sociologist Saad Nagi in response to a vast number of definitions for disability that existed, inconsistency in disability assessment, and disparity over awarding disability benefits based solely on impairments.[9] The Nagi framework provided the

**Figure 1-1.** The Nagi Disablement Framework.

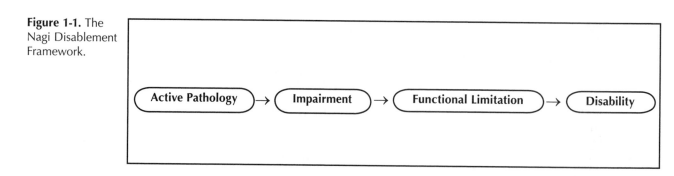

following terms and definitions as a conceptual framework linking pathology to disability (Figure 1-1):

- Active pathology
- Impairment
- Functional limitation
- Disability

In this framework, *active pathology* is defined as the interruption or interference with the body's normal processes and simultaneous body efforts to heal itself, or regain a normal state. A pathology can result from a variety of causes, including trauma and degenerative changes.[10] The pathology is often referred to as the disease itself, occurs at the cellular, tissue, or organ level, and is often the patient's medical diagnosis.[18] Medical management and physician interventions are often directed at reducing the active pathology. Examples of active pathologies include osteoporosis, Parkinson's disease, and fractures.

*Impairment* is a loss or abnormality of an anatomical, physiological, mental, or emotional nature.[10] Impairments are deviations from normal occurring at the cellular, tissue, organ, or system level. Nagi[10] described three types of impairments. The first is the disease process itself, since the disease represents a deviation from normal anatomy or physiology. Another type of impairment is the result of the pathology. These impairments comprise the signs and/or symptoms of the active pathology, or the problems remaining once the pathology has been resolved. The third type of impairment is one not caused by the pathology, but instead, it is a result of a congenital problem, such as a postural abnormality like scoliosis or club foot. In physical therapy, the two latter types are given the most consideration. Besides postural abnormalities, impairments often encountered in physical therapy practice include decreased range of motion, muscle weakness, impaired balance, and impaired sensation.

A *functional limitation* refers to an abnormality or limitation in an individual's ability to carry out a meaningful action, task, and/or activity in an efficient, competent, reasonably expected manner.[10,18] In the Nagi framework, functional limitations are experienced at the "organism" level, or as the individual functions "as a whole."[10] Functional limitations are specific to the individual and are based on the demands and activities of his or her lifestyle. This is a task or activity the individual could do prior to the onset of the pathology. Consider functional limitations as the inability to do something the person wants to do because of the existing pathology.

For example, following an elbow fracture, a 25-year-old male is limited in elbow flexion in the dominant extremity and cannot feed himself. In this example, the active pathology is the fracture, the impairment is decreased elbow range of motion, and the functional limitation is self-feeding with the dominant extremity. Now, confusion exists when the individual states he can feed himself with his non-dominant extremity. However, consideration must be given to the fact that the time it takes him to eat is increased, and he does not have good control of the utensils with the non-dominant hand. Therefore, a functional limitation still exists.

Impairments often contribute to functional limitations. For instance, an individual with limited hip range of motion (impairment) might have difficulty sitting and standing from a chair or have difficulty donning pants (both functional limitations). In addition, a patient with decreased quadriceps strength (impairment) might have difficulty ascending and descending stairs (functional limitations). When determining the effects of impairment on function, it is important to remember that functional limitations are not solely dependent on the number or severity of the impairments. Rather, an individual's normal roles and responsibilities should be given greater consideration when considering his or her functional limitations under this framework.

Consider the following two patients. Patient 1 is a 52-year-old male accountant who spends the majority of his day at his computer. Patient 2 is a 45-year-old mechanic who works with his arms elevated overhead 75% of the day. Both patients have been diagnosed with shoulder impingement syndrome and have limited shoulder range of motion while reaching overhead due to pain. Patient 1 is able to perform normal work duties, but Patient 2 is not able to work due to his inability to reach overhead without pain. For the latter patient, the impairment (decreased range of motion) is directly creating a functional limitation, whereas for Patient 1, the result of the impairment on function is less profound. Therefore, the manner in which impairments impact function is dependent more on the specific tasks the individual must carry out, rather than the number or severity of the impairments themselves.

*Disability*, the fourth aspect of the Nagi framework, is the inability or limitation in performing socially defined roles and/or tasks that would normally be expected of an individual with a similar gender or age within a given culture and/or environment.[10] The most direct way that impairments contribute to disabilities is through functional limitations.[10] Unlike functional limitations, which are patient-specific, disabilities are roles and/or tasks that have been socially defined as normal for a given population. These roles and tasks are organized by life activities including: 1) self-care, 2) home management, 3) work, 4) community activities, and 5) leisure activities.[18]

Nagi[10] provided three additional factors that influence an individual's perception of his or her degree of disability. These include: 1) the individual's situation and his or her reactions to the situation; 2) the situation and reactions of others, such as family, friends, associates, and co-workers; and 3) the presence of environmental barriers.[10] These additional factors are paralleled in the ICF (Part 2, Contextual Factors), which includes global and immediate environmental factors as well as personal factors.

In Nagi's framework, dissimilar pathologies, impairments, and functional limitations could produce similar disabilities. Furthermore, individuals with similar impairments and functional limitations might have differing degrees of disability. Consider the two patients with shoulder impingement from the last example. Both individuals have shoulder impingement syndrome (pathology), both individuals have decreased shoulder range of motion (impairment), and both individuals are limited in their ability to reach overhead due to pain (functional limitations). The patient working as a mechanic could be considered "temporarily disabled" in his ability to work (a role that is socially expected of him), whereas the accountant continues to perform the role that is normally expected of him and would not be considered to have a disability in work.

Adding to the confusion, there is often overlap between an individual's functional limitations and his or her disabilities. The reason is that a specific activity or task carried out by an individual is also a role or responsibility for an individual of his or her age, within a given environment. Consider the patient who had an elbow fracture on the dominant extremity. Self-feeding, a functional limitation, could also be considered a disability since it is a reasonable expectation of an individual his age.

In many cases, functional limitations result in compensatory behaviors. When a patient cannot perform a common task in the normal manner, he may identify another way to do it. Often, the role of the physical therapist (PT) is to assist the patient or family in identifying compensatory ways to perform normal functional tasks. In considering the case of the patient with an elbow fracture, his compensatory strategy may be feeding with his non-dominant extremity. According to the Nagi framework,[10] disability results when the patient is unable to return to what would normally be expected. When the patient identifies a compensatory strategy that is effective, efficient, and allows return to his normal socially identified role, then the patient is not considered "disabled." Recall though that his eating with the non-dominant extremity was ineffective and inefficient. Would you consider him to have a disability? The answer is, "It depends." If the patient was not able to return to some semblance of normal self-feeding with the non-dominant extremity over time and remained inefficient and ineffective, then he would be considered somewhat disabled in self-feeding. However, if the patient adapts to eating with his non-dominant extremity and is able to perform the task within a reasonable amount of time and effectiveness, then he would not have a disability.

Another consideration when correlating functional limitations and disability are co-morbidities, or prior medical conditions that complicate the patient's current problem. If the patient with the elbow fracture had previously had a stroke with resultant paralysis of the non-dominant extremity, now the functional limitation, self-feeding, is without a doubt also a disability. The patient will remain "disabled" in self-feeding until he regains normal range of motion or finds an efficient, effective way to self-feed.

As you can see, relating disability concepts is complex and confusing. Let's summarize disablement concepts according to Nagi using another example:

**Point #1: There is overlap between functional limitations and disabilities.**

- A 24-year-old male is involved in a motor vehicle accident and sustains an L2-L3 incomplete spinal cord injury. He has weakness in many of his major lower extremity muscles causing knee and ankle instability during gait. He ambulates 25' on level surfaces with an assistive device and assistance from the physical therapist.

  *Active pathology*: Incomplete L2-L3 spinal cord injury

  *Impairment*: Decreased muscle strength

  *Functional limitation*: Mobility/Gait

  *Disability*: Gait. For a healthy 24-year-old male, independent, normal ambulation for unlimited distances is an expectation.

**Point #2: Compensatory strategies, including the use of assistive devices, can allow people to overcome functional limitations, return**

to normal activities, and become "enabled," rather than "disabled."

- The patient learns to ambulate with ankle-foot orthoses and Lofstrand crutches. With the assistive devices, he can ambulate unlimited distances independently without fatiguing. Without the assistive devices, he requires assistance, and his gait is inefficient and he fatigues quickly.

  *Functional limitations*: Gait abnormalities

  *Is he disabled*? Without the assistive devices, yes. With the assistive devices, no.

**Point #3: Co-morbidities influence the way people adapt to their functional limitations and can increase the likelihood of resulting disability.**

- The patient later develops a chronic lung condition and has difficulty breathing during activities that cause exertion. He can only walk short distances with the assistive devices due to poor endurance and he uses a wheelchair for longer distances.

  *Functional limitations*: Gait abnormalities

  *Is he disabled*? Yes, when walking long distances

## The NCMRR Classification Scheme for Disability Terminology

The National Center for Medical Rehabilitation Research (NCMRR) is a branch of the National Institute of Child Health and Human Development of the National Institutes of Health (NIH). In the early 1990s, Congress directed the NIH to establish a special committee to provide guidance to the NCMRR for rehabilitation research initiatives. This special committee was called the National Advisory Board on Medical Rehabilitation Research (NABMRR). The goal was for the Advisory Board to assist the NIH in extending the same excellence to rehabilitation science research that was extended to biological science research. The hope was to improve research related to improving function and enhancing quality of life for people with disabilities.[19]

Acknowledging previously developed disablement frameworks, the NABMRR indicated that none of them suited their intent to describe the role of rehabilitation in improving function and quality of life. Consequently, the NABMRR also identified five domains relevant to rehabilitation—pathophysiolo-

gy, impairment, functional limitation, disability, and societal limitation.[19] Definitions provided for these domains are as follows[19(pp5,23-25)]:

- *Pathophysiology*: An interruption of, or interference with normal physiological and developmental processes or structures; occurs at the cellular or tissue level
- *Impairment*: A loss or abnormality of cognitive, emotional, physiological, or anatomical structure or function; occurs in the organ or organ system
- *Functional Limitation*: Restriction or lack of ability to perform the task designated; abnormal function of an organism
- *Disability*: Inability or limitation in performance of tasks, activities, and roles at levels typically expected within a given social context; occurs at the level of the individual
- *Societal Limitation*: Restriction due to social policy or barriers, physical or attitudinal, limiting the fulfillment of roles or denying access to services and opportunities associated with full societal participation (ie, vocation, housing, health care, etc.) occurs at the societal level, or how the individual functions within society

In putting forth this framework, the NABMRR suggested a research plan in which these domains would serve as "five overlapping domains of research that are relevant to studying disability."[19(p9)] In developing the framework, the NABMRR suggested examples of research under each of the domains.

In summary, the WHO, Nagi, and NCMRR have provided frameworks for defining disability terminology and examining the relationship between disease, impairments, limitations in function, disability, and function within society. In addition, these frameworks provide a mechanism for allowing clinicians and researchers to be aware of the impact of disease on an individual's day-to-day life and overall function within society. Consideration of a disablement model when working with patients helps therapists to realize more complex functional and social issues that patients face due to the health condition, disease, or injury.

## Disablement and Physical Therapy

Individuals in need of physical therapy services often have a disease or injury with resulting impairments. It is our responsibility to understand how these impairments affect their day-to-day activities—in a variety of settings and situations. In 1989, Jette[20] put forth the idea of PTs using a disablement framework, primarily for patient diagnosis and classification. He explained how the ICIDH (now called the ICF) provided a structure for classifying information gathered during a physical therapy examination that is pertinent for our diagnosis and treatment of patients. For example, following the physical therapy examination, the PT would not only document the patient's medical diagnosis (which may or may not be determined by the physician) but would also provide the "impairment diagnosis," the "diagnosis of physical disability," and the "handicap diagnosis."[20(p88)] Providing structure to the examination in this manner would allow for the provision of information on the *consequences* of disease (rather than the disease alone), which tends to be a primary focus of physical therapy intervention. In his opinion, a disablement framework was a necessary step toward formation of a scientific basis for the profession.[20]

In 1991, Guccione[21] reported limitations in using the ICIDH in physical therapy and recommended the use of the Nagi framework. In supporting the Nagi framework, he identified reasons that it was more useful than the ICIDH for PTs. Reasons included: 1) the degree of functional limitation was based not only on the extent of the impairment, but also on the individual's normal roles and responsibilities; 2) the idea that disability occurs after a period of being unable to compensate for a functional limitation; 3) the effect(s) of the individual's attitude, others' perceptions, and environmental barriers on disability; and 4) the importance of identifying impairments that are causing the functional limitation. Nevertheless, Guccione[21] also indicated problems with the Nagi framework and identified ways that it could be modified to further meet the needs of PTs. These included "expanding the concept of disease" to include syndromes and lesions, considering services that the patient had already received, and identifying "personal characteristics that are either known or hypothesized to affect disablement."[21(pp12-13)] Guccione's expanded version of Nagi's framework was adopted for use in *The Guide to Physical Therapist Practice* to serve as a framework for physical therapist practice and diagnosis.[18]

In 1994, Verbrugge and Jette[5] discussed disablement as a "process," rather than a delineated pathway from pathology to disability. These authors indicated that the pathway to disability was influenced by non-medical factors such as social, environmental, and psychological factors. They also reported the disablement process was the "functional consequences over time and the factors that affect their direction, pace, and patterns of change."[5(p3)] In addition, these authors discussed: 1) the influence of risk factors, or predisposing factors that may prompt disablement; 2) the aim of interventions, like physical therapy, to reduce disability; and 3) the notion of intrinsic and external factors that exacerbate disability.[5] These include things like the individual's or others' attitudes and existing environmental barriers. Keeping with the Nagi framework as the main pathway from pathology to disability, yet realizing facilitating and inhibiting factors to the disablement process, Verbrugge and

Jette[5] proposed an alternate sociomedial model suggesting the influence of environmental demands and individual capabilities on disability.

More recently, Jette[22] again identified a need for a common language in physical therapy clinical practice and research. In this article, traditional frameworks were discussed and the author concluded that the "ICF holds great promise to provide a synthesis of earlier models of disablement and to provide the rehabilitation disciplines with a universal language with which to discuss disability."[22(p733)] Nevertheless, more work needs to be done to blend disablement into areas of physical therapy practice including terminology, examination, evaluation, and research.

# Integrating Disablement and Documentation

*Documentation*, otherwise known as medical record-keeping, has been defined as "any entry into the patient-client record, such as a(n) consultation report, initial examination report, progress note, flow sheet/checklist, that identifies the care/service provided, re-examination, or summation of care."[18(p703)] Redgate and Foto[23] indicated that complete documentation also includes the physician prescription(s) and certification(s), communication with other care providers, copies of exercise programs or patient instructions, as well as any other care providers' notes or comments that support the interventions provided.

As you have read, there is a need in physical therapy for consistency in terminology for practice, reimbursement, and research. This begins by way of consistency in our documentation, since our "notes" are the sole record of the episode of care provided to each patient or client. Using *The Guide to Physical Therapist Practice* is one way to begin using consistent terminology. However, disablement terminology, especially those terms linking impairment, function, and interventions, is also a necessary element for our documentation. In more traditional physical therapy documentation formats, however, these links are often omitted or implied, resulting in an unclear or inadequate picture of the patient. Disablement terminology in documenting patient status, interventions, and progress provides a better picture in terms of how the disease (or injury) and intervention(s) affect the patient's functional status and participation in his or her normal roles and responsibilities.

Disablement concepts can be integrated into the initial examination through measuring and documenting impairments and function. The physical therapy examination will illuminate the individual's impairments. These are often limitations in range of motion, strength, balance, etc. The examination, however, must go beyond the impairment level to determine how the patient's ability to function has been compromised. This includes documenting the patient's ability or inability to perform meaningful tasks such as hygiene or dressing, manage the home environment, and participate in normal life situations such as work or school-related functions. By understanding and documenting an individual's impairments as well as limitations in his or her normal life roles, we can better communicate the consequences of the disease or injury. Further, documentation must specifically explain the relationship between impairments and function.

Additionally, the physical therapy interventions are often aimed at reducing the individual's impairments. For example, we teach patients to perform range of motion and strengthening exercises. In doing these exercises, we hope to not only reduce impairments, but also to improve function and reduce disability. Documentation should describe the effects of intervention on not only impairments but also on function.

In summary, the physical therapy examination should include examination of impairments as well as function and provide a picture of how the patient's impairments relate, or cause his or her limitations in function and disability. Additionally, documentation should show that physical therapy interventions are bringing about substantial changes in impairments,

*Ways to integrate disablement into our clinical documentation:*

- Document impairments, functional problems, and limitations in life tasks and situations.
- Describe the relationship between the impairments and functional deficits, eg, how a range of motion or strength limitation is preventing a functional task or participation in a normal role.
- Describe the effects of treatment on impairments and function, eg, joint mobilizations and stretching have increased lower extremity range of motion, allowing the patient to better ascend and descend stairs, sit, and ambulate.

function, and disability. As you will read in subsequent chapters, documentation serves many purposes, such as maintaining data collected and providing information to insurance companies. There are many styles and formats for physical therapy records. Regardless of the style that you are using, your documentation should use consistent disablement terminology.

## Review Questions

1. In your own words, define disablement. Give an example of how a person can be disabled according to the definition you provided.

2. Compare and contrast the definition of "health" using the biomedical and biopsychosocial models.

3. List reasons for the development of disablement frameworks.

4. List the major disablement frameworks.

5. Complete the table on the following page using terminology from the ICF, Nagi, and NCMRR frameworks using the following terms: pathology, pathophysiology, impairment, functional limitation, disability, activity limitation, participation restriction, and societal limitation.

| | ICF | Nagi | NCMRR |
|---|---|---|---|
| A patient's medical diagnosis | | | |
| Loss or abnormality of an individual's anatomy or physiology | | | |
| Difficulties or limitations that are encountered when an individual attempts to complete a task | | | |
| Problems an individual faces while involved in life situations | | | |
| Encompasses impairments and limitations in abilities to carry out socially acceptable tasks | | | |
| Unable to carry out a task that would be socially appropriate for an individual | | | |

6. What is the difference between:
   a. ADL and IADL?
   b. Functional limitation and disability?
   c. Activity limitation and participation restriction?
   d. The Functioning and Disability and Contextual Factors components of the ICF?
   e. Positive and negative aspects of disease according to the ICF?

7. How are impairments and functional limitations related?

8. How are impairments, functional limitations, and disability related?

9. How are deviations from normal body structure and function scored using the ICF?

10. How are activities and participation scored using the ICF?

11. What factors affect activities and participation? Give an example of a patient you might see clinically.

12. What is the WHO-FIC? What is it comprised of? Why is it recommended?

13. What disablement frameworks have been proposed for use in physical therapy? How would these be used?

14. Identify barriers to integrating concepts of disablement into physical therapy.

15. How should disablement be reflected in documentation?

16. The Nagi framework implies that pathology leads to impairment. Do you think impairment can lead to pathology? Why or why not? If so, give an example.

# Application Exercises

I. Determine whether the following is (are) pathology (P), impairment (I), activity limitation (AL), or participation restriction (PR) according to the ICF.

_____ elbow flexion contracture

_____ right hip osteoarthritis

_____ A 48-year-old male requires a wheelchair for community mobility and can self-propel 200' on level surfaces prior to fatigue; requires assist for community mobility

_____ Opening a heavy door

_____ A patient with impaired mobility is unable to go to the grocery store due to lack of a wheelchair ramp at the grocery store entrance

_____ decreased shoulder range of motion

_____ emphysema

_____ congenital hip dysplasia

_____ A 55-year-old male is unable to open a jar due weakness following a cerebrovascular accident

_____ A 65-year-old female with rheumatoid arthritis uses a button hook to dress due to hand weakness and deformity

II. Determine whether the following is (are) pathology (P), impairment (I), functional limitation (FL), or disability (D) according to the Nagi framework.

_____ right transtibial amputation

_____ knee flexion contracture

_____ A 52-year-old male requires minimal assist for household ambulation

_____ A patient with impaired mobility is unable to leave his house due to lack of a wheelchair ramp at the house entrance

_____ poor balance

_____ poor endurance

_____ A 35-year-old male is unable to work on an assembly line in a meat packing plant due to a shoulder injury

_____ emphysema

_____ A 65-year-old female with rheumatoid arthritis uses a button hook to dress due to hand weakness and deformity

_____ A 20-year-old male uses a sliding board and moderate assistance to transfer bed to wheelchair following a spinal cord injury

III. From the list in Part II, which could be functional limitations and disabilities?

IV. Read the following two scenarios and determine the patient's:
- pathology
- functional limitations
- activity limitations
- participation restrictions
- environmental factors/facilitators
- environmental factors/barriers
- *possible* personal factors (facilitators or barriers) that could potentially effect the degree of disability

1. You are working with a 10-year-old female in the school system. Her medical diagnosis is spastic diplegia. You have been working on ambulating up and down the stairs (which she can perform with minimal assist of 1 and a quad cane and handrail) and increasing the speed of her gait. At the present time, she leaves her classes early so that she can make it to the next one on time and she uses the elevator rather than the stairs.

2. Your patient is a 35-year-old who sustained a traumatic, closed head injury in a motorcycle accident. He is confused and disoriented and he requires constant supervision for his safety. He can perform ADLs with supervision and occasional verbal cues. He can walk and get in and out of bed with supervision. He can also ascend and descend stairs with supervision. He has not returned to work as a radiologic technician since his injury. He has family that can provide 24-hour supervision.

# References

1. Law M. *Evidence-Based Rehabilitation: A Guide to Practice*. Thorofare, NJ: SLACK Incorporated; 2002.
2. National Center for Health Statistics. NCHS definitions [Centers for Disease Control Web site]. 2005. Available at: http://www.cdc.gov/nchs/datawh/nchsdefs/healthcondition.htm. Accessed March 1, 2006.
3. World Health Organization. WHO definition of health. Official Records of the World Health Organization: Preamble to the Constitution of the World Health Organization as adopted by the International Conference (New York, 19-22 June 1946) by the Representatives of the 61 states. 2003;No. 2:100. Available at: http://www.who.int/about/definition/en/print.html. Accessed March 1, 2006.

4. World Health Organization. *World Health Organization Family of International Classifications*. Available at: http://www.who.int/classifications/en/WHOFICFamily.pdf. Accessed April 26, 2006.

5. Verbrugge LM, Jette AM. The disablement process. *Soc Sci Med*. 1994;38(1):1-14.

6. Sokolow J, Silson JE, Taylor EJ, Anderson ET, Rusk HA. A method for the functional evaluation of disability. *Arch Phys Med Rehabil*. 1959;40(Oct):421-8.

7. Townsend P. *The Disabled in Society*. London, England: Greater London Association for the Disabled; 1967.

8. Gresham GE, Labi MLC. Functional assessment instruments currently available for documenting outcomes in rehabilitation medicine. In: Granger CV, Gresham GE, eds. *Functional Assessment in Rehabilitation Medicine*. Baltimore, MD: Williams and Wilkins; 1984:65-85.

9. Pope A, Tarlov A, eds. *Disability in America: Toward a National Agenda for Prevention*. Washington, DC: National Academy Press; 1991.

10. Nagi S. Disability concepts revisited: implications for prevention. In: Pope AM, Tarlov AR, eds. *Disability in America: Toward a National Agenda for Prevention*. Washington, D.C.: National Academy Press; 1991:309-27.

11. World Health Organization. *International Classification of Functioning, Disability and Health*. Available at: http://whqlibdoc.who.int/publications/2001/9241545429.pdf. Accessed March 29, 2006.

12. World Health Organization. *ICF Classification Hypertext Version*. Available at: http://www3.who.int/icf/onlinebrowser/icf.cfm?parentlevel=1&childlevel=2&itemslevel=1&ourdimension=s&ourchapter=0&ourblock=0&our2nd=0&our3rd=0&our4th=0. Accessed April 6, 2006.

13. World Health Organization. *ICF Checklist*. 2003. Available at: http://www3.who.int/icf/checklist/icf-checklist.pdf. Accessed February 1, 2006.

14. Okochi J, Utsunomiya S, Takahashi T. Health measurement using the ICF: test-retest reliability study of ICF codes and qualifiers in geriatric care [BioMed Central]. *Health and Quality of Life Outcomes* [serial online]. 3(46). Available at: http://www.hqlo.com/content/3/1/46. Accessed February 19, 2007.

15. Jette AM, Haley SM, Kooyoomjian JT. Are the ICF activity and participation dimensions distinct. *J Rehabil Med*. 2003;35:145-9.

16. Harris JE, MacDermid JC, Roth J. The International Classification of Functioning as an explanatory model of health after distal radius fracture: a cohort study. *Health and Quality of Life Outcomes* [serial online]. 2005;3(73). Available at: http://www.hqlo.com/content/3/1/73. Accessed April 26, 2006.

17. World Health Organization. *International Classification of Health Interventions*. 2006. Available at: http://www.who.int/classifications/ichi/en/index.html. Accessed April 6, 2006.

18. American Physical Therapy Association. *The Guide to Physical Therapist Practice*. Alexandria, VA: APTA; 2001.

19. National Advisory Board on Medical Rehabilitation Research. *Research Plan for the National Center for Medical Rehabilitation Research*. Rockville, MD: National Institutes of Health; 1993. NIH Publication No. 93-3509.

20. Jette AM. Diagnosis and classification by physical therapists: a special communication. *Phys Ther*. 1989;69(11):87-9.

21. Guccione A. Physical therapy diagnosis and the relationship between impairments and function. *Phys Ther*. 1991;71(7):10-4.

22. Jette AM. Toward a common language for function, disability, and health. *Phys Ther*. 2006;86(5):726-34.

23. Redgate N, Foto M. Pay by the rules: avoid Medicare audits and reduce payment denials with a sound strategy and proper documentation. *Physical Therapy Products*. 2003;October/November:28-30.

## Chapter 2

# Reasons for Documenting in Physical Therapy

*Mia Erickson, PT, EdD, CHT, ATC; Rebecca McKnight, PT, MS*

## Chapter Objectives

Upon completion of this chapter, the reader will be able to:

1. List reasons for documenting in physical therapy.
2. List components of the Patient/Client Management Model that are included in documentation.
3. Explain how interim and discharge notes should be related to initial documentation.
4. Explain how documentation demonstrates clinical problem solving.
5. Examine the relationship between reimbursement and documentation.
6. Describe criteria for medical necessity and skilled care.
7. Differentiate between skilled care and maintenance therapy.
8. List situations when maintenance therapy can be considered skilled care.
9. Explain the PTA's role in the clinical decision-making process.

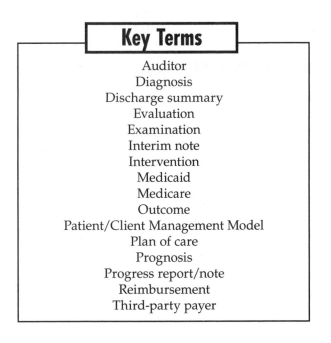

### Key Terms

Auditor
Diagnosis
Discharge summary
Evaluation
Examination
Interim note
Intervention
Medicaid
Medicare
Outcome
Patient/Client Management Model
Plan of care
Prognosis
Progress report/note
Reimbursement
Third-party payer

```
┌─────────────────────────┐
│   Key Abbreviations     │
├─────────────────────────┤
│         APTA            │
│         CMS             │
│         PT              │
│         PTA             │
└─────────────────────────┘
```

## Introduction

In the 1960s, medical records existed to: 1) provide a legal record of care, 2) facilitate communication among health care providers, and 3) serve as a source of information for clinical research.[1] In the 1970s, documentation became a requirement for reimbursement by government agencies such as Medicare and Medicaid. Medicare began requiring rehabilitation facilities to not only maintain documentation, but also to submit the records to be reviewed by Medicare auditors. Auditors reviewed documentation to determine if physical therapy services provided to Medicare beneficiaries met requirements for reimbursement.[1] Since then, documentation has become a reimbursement requirement for most third-party payers. A third-party payer is an insurance company or other organization/agency that pays for services provided to a patient. Many of these payers are also conducting audits to determine if the documentation meets reimbursement requirements. Today, physical therapy documentation is scrutinized more than ever by third-party payers.

In addition to reimbursement, there are legal and ethical obligations to maintain accurate medical records. For example, there are federal and state laws that mandate recording medical or health care provided to an individual. Finally, facilities and organizations providing components of patient/client management often employ documentation policies and procedures beyond state and federal law.

## Record Patient/Client Management

The Patient/Client Management Model, described in detail in *The Guide to Physical Therapist Practice*,[2] outlines components of care provided to a patient once he or she has entered into the physical therapy system. These essential components include examination, evaluation, diagnosis, prognosis, and intervention.[2] Following the final component, intervention, patient/client management will lead to an outcome. This is the end result of patient/client management. The term *outcome* is defined as "the impact of physical therapy interventions on the following domains: pathology; impairments; functional limitations; disabilities; risk reduction/prevention; health, wellness, and fitness; societal resources; and patient/client satisfaction."[2(p43)]

---

*Reasons for documenting*
- Record patient/client management
- Demonstrate clinical problem-solving
- Reimbursement
- Provide proof of medical necessity
- Provide proof of and need for skilled care
- Communication
- Outcomes research
- Legal action

One of the primary reasons for documenting in physical therapy is to maintain a record of patient/client management that reflects the patient's entire episode of care. The initial encounter is recorded by documenting the examination findings, the evaluation, the patient's physical therapy diagnosis, the prognosis, and the plan of care.[3] This initial documentation reflects the patient's status upon entering the physical therapy system, and it serves as the baseline to which future measurements are compared. The initial encounter is performed and recorded by the physical therapist (PT).

Subsequent patient encounters, visits, or treatment sessions are documented in *interim notes*. Interim notes are also called treatment encounter notes, daily notes, or progress notes. These interim notes are written to maintain ongoing records of subjective and objective data; specific intervention(s) provided; results of the intervention(s); the patient's response(s) to the interventions in terms of impairments, function, and disability; changes (or need for changes) in the plan of care; need for referral to another practitioner; and plans for subsequent treatment/intervention.[3] They are also required to support what was billed for a given date of service.

The final encounter with the patient is recorded by documenting a discharge note, or discharge summary, describing the patient's final status, outcome, and plans for ongoing treatment, such as a home exercise program.[3]

## Demonstrate Clinical Problem-Solving

At each patient encounter, PTs will have to go through a clinical problem-solving process to manage each patient's condition. This clinical problem-solving

| Table 2-1 | |
|---|---|
| *Parallels Between Problem Solving and Patient/Client Management* | |
| *Steps associated with problem solving include[4]:* | *Steps involved in clinical problem-solving in patient/client management include:* |
| 1. Recognize a problem | 1. Recognize deviations from normal body structure and function and determine reasons for these deviations |
| 2. Represent the problem | 2. Create a patient problem list and determine the physical therapy diagnosis |
| 3. Devise or choose a plan | 3. Determine a physical therapy plan of care that includes specific interventions |
| 4. Execute the plan | 4. Carry out the intervention plan |
| 5. Evaluate the solution | 5. Determine the patient's response to the intervention |

process reflects steps associated with traditional problem-solving skills (Table 2-1).

This clinical problem-solving process must be reflected in the patient's record from the initial encounter to discharge. Physical therapy documentation should delineate the clinician's problem-solving and clinical judgment.[5-7] Any individual who does not know the patient should be able to read the physical therapy record and identify the patient's physical therapy problems and steps taken to specifically address each problem. In addition, the record must reflect the clinician's determination of intervention adequacy. This may be accomplished through ongoing documentation of the patient's status and his or her response to the interventions being provided. Documentation should reflect logical decisions and sound judgment by explicitly linking data collected, patient problems, goals, interventions, changes in patient status, changes in intervention, and discharge status. Documentation that demonstrates problem solving also improves the provider's credibility with third-party payers.[8]

Following the initial encounter, both the PT and the physical therapist assistant (PTA) must use clinical problem solving throughout the episode of care. In addition, both the PT and PTA are responsible for assuring that clinical problem solving is reflected in the medical records. For example:

- **PT role**: Data collected during the initial examination are reflected in the evaluation, diagnosis, prognosis, and plan of care. For instance, patient problem lists and goals written by the PT reflect impairments and functional deficits identified during the initial examination.

- **PT role**: The plan of care includes physical therapy interventions aimed at reducing the identified impairments and functional deficits.

- **PT and PTA role**: Collect pertinent subjective patient data at follow-up therapy sessions and record it in interim notes. Subjective data often gathered include: 1) asking the patient about his or her response to a previous treatment, 2) inquiring about adherence with a home exercise program, or 3) asking the patient if the treatment has improved function. When asking a patient if the treatment has improved function, clinicians should refer back to the initial documentation so that inquiries and questions directed to the patient can be specific to his or her prior status.

- **PT and PTA role**: Collect pertinent objective patient data at follow-up therapy sessions and record it in interim notes. Objective data include tests and measures such as range of motion (ROM) measurements, strength measurements, girth or volumetric measurements of edema, etc. In most cases, it is important to identify and perform the same tests and measurements performed during the initial examination so that you can identify changes in status since the initial examination.

- **PT and PTA role**: Make frequent comparisons between the patient's current and prior status for both subjective and objective data and document changes. Changes in patient status are stated explicitly and brought to the reader's attention, rather than assuming the reader will identify the change. Changes in status are supported by making specific reference to objective data found in the chart. For example, "The patient's range of motion for the left shoulder improved 20 degrees in 1 week." *or* "The patient ambulated 150' today compared to 50' two days ago."

- **PT and PTA role**: Changes in patient status elicit changes in the plan of care (Both the PT and PTA recognize changes in patient status; PT changes the plan of care).

Consistency between the initial, interim, and discharge documentation makes it easier to identify and follow the clinical problem-solving process. Ongoing documentation of subjective remarks and objective findings tell the story of the patient's response to treatment. In addition, consistency between initial and subsequent documentation makes it easier for the clinician(s) to identify progress, or lack thereof. Finally, comparing current data to that gathered during the initial examination allows the PT to easily update goals and interventions as needed.

# Reimbursement

Third-party payers are very interested in our records of patient data. Consider the following example:

## Example 1

Imagine that you are a PT working in a small, outpatient private practice. For the last 6 weeks, you have been working with a 35-year-old male who was recently involved in a motorcycle accident. In the accident, he sustained a mild concussion and multiple left lower extremity fractures to the femur and tibia. Initially, he was unable to bear weight through the extremity and required a wheelchair for mobility. He had significant loss in range of motion and strength. Also, he was unable to perform independent self-care, normal home/community mobility including ambulation, and his usual work activities. Since the initial visit, he has been making excellent progress and is now able to walk using one crutch, weight bearing as tolerated through the left lower extremity, and he has resumed most of his normal activities of daily living. After seeing him for 14 visits, it is brought to your attention that his insurance requires authorization for visits occurring after the initial 15. In order to have additional therapy services approved, you must submit adequate documentation showing evidence of: 1) the patient's progress, and 2) medical necessity of continued treatment. Continuation of physical therapy benefits is based largely on how well you have objectively documented his improvement in impairments and function. It can prove that he needs further care that will benefit his condition.

Reimbursement from third-party payers is directly linked with documentation and its ability to show the need for physical therapy services provided. In fact, an American Physical Therapy Association (APTA) House of Delegates Policy (06-94-16-28) for provision of physical therapy services within the healthcare system stated, "Reimbursement for physical therapy services should occur only when adequate physical therapy documentation exists which is consistent with APTA guidelines. Such documentation should support the need for physical therapy services."[9] Communication with third-party payers through appropriate documentation has been determined to be the "key to securing reimbursement."[8] The Centers for Medicare and Medicaid Services (CMS) as well as other third-party payers have provided documentation requirements to maximize reimbursement and minimize payment denials.

# Provide Proof of Medical Necessity

Physical therapy documentation must provide evidence that services provided to a patient are both medically necessary and require skills of trained personnel. Recent language in documentation requirements put forth by CMS indicated that "medically necessary" is analogous to "reasonable and necessary." Services or supplies that are reasonable and necessary meet the following criteria[10]:

1. They are proper, consistent with, and needed for the diagnosis or treatment of a medical condition.

2. They meet the standards of good medical practice in the local area to be safe, specific, and effective in treating a patient's condition.

3. They require skills of a trained therapist or must be performed under supervision of a trained therapist (this is also known as "skilled service"—see next section).

4. They will lead to a change in the patient's condition within a reasonable amount of time.

5. They include an appropriate amount, frequency, and duration that are reasonable under acceptable standards of practice.

6. They are not mainly for the convenience of the patient or health care provider.

PTs determine whether an intervention is medically necessary (or reasonable and necessary) based on their knowledge of the patient's pathology or disease process, familiarity with physical therapy interventions and alternatives, awareness of the standard of practice for treating that pathology, and the best available research evidence.[11]

In proving medical necessity, each physical therapy problem must be addressed in the plan of care.

In addition, documentation must demonstrate how the specific interventions are aimed at reducing a specific, documented pathology, impairment, functional deficit, and/or limitation in normal activity. Documentation should indicate that the patient is progressing as expected. Documentation showing objective, comparative data throughout the episode of care, and therapeutic interventions with resulting functional improvement, can both serve as evidence of patient progress. Documenting remaining functional deficits and benefits of continued intervention will then support the need for further treatment due to medical necessity. Finally, the patient should have good potential for improvement within a reasonable amount of time. Documentation showing no improvement in patient status can also provide a rationale for discontinuing physical therapy services.

At regular intervals throughout the episode of care, the PT must provide proof that interventions continue to be medically necessary. This can be accomplished through formal re-examinations and re-evaluations or an informal assessment of patient status. Unlike informal assessments, formal re-examinations and re-evaluations have a separate procedure code and associated fee that can be billed because of the increased time requirement to complete; however, some third-party payers have rules as to when and if it will be reimbursed. Regardless, there must be regular updates to the patient's plan of care that address goals set on the initial evaluation, and these updates must provide proof of ongoing medical necessity of care being provided.

Federal rules and regulations, state law, third-party payers, or the facility will dictate the frequency of these re-examinations or reassessments. For example, the outpatient clinic where you work may require a re-evaluation of the patient's goals every six visits, or the inpatient facility might require you to address the patient's goals every week.

## Provide Proof of Skilled Care

In addition to being medically necessary (or reasonable and necessary), documentation must reflect the patient's need for skilled care. *Skilled care,* otherwise known as skilled services, has been defined as a type of health care given when a patient needs management, observation, or evaluation by trained nurses or rehabilitation staff.[12] In order for an intervention to be considered "skilled," a patient must have a pathology or injury that results in a documented physical or functional limitation and requires a sophisticated and complex intervention that can only be carried out by a licensed PT or PTA. This intervention requires the unique judgment and/or skill of a trained individual for both safety and effectiveness. As with reasonable and necessary, a skilled intervention is targeted at reducing a specific impairment or functional deficit and is related specifically to the plan of care.[13] According to the APTA, documentation that shows clinical decision making and problem solving lends further support to prove interventions are skilled.[13]

Documentation of a medical condition alone is not a factor for determining whether or not the patient requires skilled services. For example, consider a patient with multiple sclerosis. Only documenting the presence of the pathology does not qualify the patient for skilled services, but documenting recent declines in function may qualify the patient for skilled services.

Services that are not skilled are often known as unskilled and are considered palliative or maintenance. Maintenance services are those that are routine, promote the general health of the patient, "maintain" the patient's present status, and do not require the unique and complex skills of a PT or PTA for safety and/or effectiveness.[10] An example is performance of an exercise program for a patient who wants to maintain motion or strength achieved in a formal physical therapy program. Maintenance therapy services can be provided by a non-licensed individual, such as the patient himself, a family member, or caregiver who has had training from a skilled professional. Maintenance services are generally not reimbursed by Medicare or many other third-party payers.[11]

There are several instances when maintenance services are considered skilled. These include[10]:

1. When the PT or PTA works with the patient and/or family to provide instruction of a home exercise program prior to discharge from a facility or outpatient therapy program.

2. When a PT evaluates a patient and establishes a home exercise maintenance program when no other services are provided (Example: A patient with osteoarthritis is referred for evaluation and establishment of an aquatic therapy program. Following the evaluation, the PT works with the patient for two to three sessions to increase the patient's independence in performing the aquatic program).

3. When the patient's safety may be jeopardized as in cases where the patient has either a complex, unpredictable medical situation, multiple co-morbidities complicating his or her situation, or when the result of the situation or intervention is unpredictable. This rule may apply to a patient who requires routine ROM exercises but the presence of unstable or recent fractures allows the intervention to be considered skilled care. Of course, documentation must support the rationale for the skilled intervention in these situations.

## Communication

Records of patient data are important to other individuals involved in the patient's care. Other health care providers including physicians, nurses, occupational and speech therapists, and case managers are often interested in a patient's status, and these individuals often need to refer to the physical therapy documentation. For example, in an inpatient hospital setting, a physician might be interested in how safely a patient can ambulate when deciding whether or not to send the patient home. Nurses might be interested in a patient's ability to transfer in and out of bed, and case managers often need to identify equipment needs or return to work status. Therefore, documenting patient data serves as a useful tool for facilitating communication across disciplines.

In addition to interdisciplinary communication, documentation serves as a reference for individuals that will be working with your patients in your absence due to vacation, illness, or days off. Clearly written notes will help those that are filling in to provide appropriate care much more efficiently. Transfer of physical therapy services is also quite common, and well-written notes can facilitate efficient transfer of care from one setting to another. Finally, it is important to consider the role that documentation plays within the PT/PTA relationship. Good documentation practices by both the PT and the PTA are imperative as a component of the communication necessary between the two providers to ensure legal, ethical, and consistent physical therapy services across the episode of care.

## Outcomes Research

Accurate records of patient data also aid in our ability to analyze and study patient outcomes. Outcomes research is a growing area in physical therapy that is necessary for reimbursement and to establish evidence for physical therapy interventions (see Chapter 10).

## Legal Action

Medical records are legal documents, and any entries made into the medical record become part of that legal document. For this reason, it is important that your documentation is accurate, legible, and depicts the patient's condition and the intervention appropriately and completely. Be aware that a patient's medical records can be subpoenaed and used as evidence in a variety of legal matters. These include motor vehicle accidents, worker's compensation or disability claims, and malpractice suits brought against you or other health care providers.

In malpractice lawsuits, documentation is the clinician's first line of defense.[14] Notes that are "clear, objective, thorough, and relevant make plaintiff's allegations of negligence more difficult to prove."[15(p2)] Good documentation can prevent a lawsuit, but poor documentation can be "powerful evidence in support of a suit, even when the accusations are frivolous."[6(p30)] Consider the following as a rule of thumb: If it isn't documented, it didn't happen. Following the guidelines for documentation in this text, recommendations set forth by the APTA, state and federal laws, government agencies' (ie, Medicare and Medicaid) policies, and facility policies can help protect you if you become involved in a malpractice lawsuit.

---

## Review Questions

1. List reasons why physical therapists and physical therapist assistants document.

2. Explain how a physical therapist's clinical problem solving can be reflected in his/her documentation.

3. Explain how reimbursement is related to documentation.

4. What are the criteria for determining if a treatment is medically necessary (or reasonable and necessary)?

5. Is maintenance therapy reimbursed by insurance companies or third-party payers? If so, when?

6. How can a PTA assist in the following tasks:

   a. Demonstrate problem solving in documentation?

   b. Gather subjective and/or objective data?

   c. Determine medical necessity or need for skilled care?

7. How does the patient's rehabilitation potential, ie, prognosis for improvement, influence his or her need for medically necessary, skilled care?

## Application Exercises

Read through the following scenarios and decide if the treatment would be considered maintenance or skilled. Give an explanation for your answer. If you choose maintenance, what are some things that you should do to initiate discontinuing treatment?

1. You are working with a patient in a nursing home who has severe Alzheimer's disease. Every afternoon, you take her for a walk through the hallways, around the building. She demonstrates weakness in her right ankle, and there is a foot slap during the contact phase of gait. She can control it if given verbal cueing. You have been working with her for a month and you are not seeing any follow through from one session to the next, and she has not progressed her distance in the last 2 weeks.

2. You have been doing some work for a home health agency in the evenings to make some extra money. The patient you are currently seeing has not shown improvement in the last week or so. She is an 85-year-old lady with Parkinson's disease who lives with her daughter. You are considering discharge when one day the patient's daughter tells you that her mother enjoys having you come in and they really believe that you are helping.

3. You are working in a skilled nursing unit and you are assigned a patient who requires maximum assist for transfers and cannot participate in therapy due to lethargy and confusion. Every day, you do PROM to all extremities and transfer the patient to the bedside chair.

4. You are working in an outpatient physical therapy clinic with a patient who has a frozen shoulder. She has been participating in therapy for about 6 weeks. During that time, she has made a substantial amount of progress. Recently, her ROM has started to plateau. The patient attends therapy twice a week for stretching and joint mobilizations.

5. You are working on gait training with a patient who had a right CVA and has resultant left hemiplegia. While ambulating, you provide tactile verbal and cueing to the quadriceps to achieve full knee extension in late swing. The patient can respond to your cues about 50% of the time. This has improved over the last week.

## References

1. Inaba M, Jones SL. Medical documentation for third-party payers. *Phys Ther.* 1977;57(7):791-4.

2. American Physical Therapy Association. *The Guide to Physical Therapist Practice.* Alexandria, VA: APTA; 2001.

3. American Physical Therapy Association. Guidelines: Physical Therapy Documentation of Patient/Client Management. Available at: http://www.apta.org/AM/Template.cfm?Section=Policies_and_Bylaws&TEMPLATE=/CM/ContentDisplay.cfm&CONTENTID=31688. Accessed July 7, 2007.

4. Beyer BK. *Practical Strategies for the Teaching of Thinking.* Boston, MA: Allyn and Bacon; 1987.

5. Arriaga R. Liability awareness. Stories from the front: documentation and clinical decision making: a real-life scenario illustrates some basic risk-management principles. *PT Magazine.* 2002;10(5):46-9.

6. Lewis DK. Do the write thing: document everything. *PT Magazine.* 2002;10(7):30-34.

7. Redgate N, Foto M. Pay by the rules: avoid Medicare audits and reduce payment denials with a sound strategy and proper documentation. *Physical Therapy Products.* 2003;October/November:28-30.

8. Baeten AM. Documentation: the reviewer perspective. *Topics in Geriatric Rehabilitation.* 1997;13(1):14-22.

9. American Physical Therapy Association House of Delegates. Principles for delivering physical therapy services within the health care system HOD 06-94-16-28 [APTA Web site]. Available at: http://www.apta.org/governance/HOD/policies/HoDPolicies/Section_I/LEGISLATION/HOD_06941628. Accessed February 11, 2004.

10. Centers for Medicare and Medicaid Services. Medicare Benefit Policy Manual. Centers for Medicare and Medicaid Services Web site; Internet-Only Manuals: 2006. Publication No. 100-02, Ch. 15-Section 220.

11. Moorhead JF, Clifford J. Determining medical necessity of outpatient physical therapy services. *Am J Med Qual.* 1992;7(3):81-4.

12. Centers for Medicare and Medicaid Services. Medicare glossary. Available at: http://www.medicare.gov/Glossary/Search.asp. Accessed May 18, 2006.

13. American Physical Therapy Association. Defensible documentation. Available at: http://www.apta.org/AM/Template.cfm?Section=Home&NAVMENUID=2505&CONTENTID=37071&DIRECTLISTCOMBOIND=D&TEMPLATE=/MembersOnly.cfm. Accessed July 28, 2007.

14. Schunk CR. Liability awareness. Advice for the new physical therapist: here are some keys to avoiding risk once you've made the transition from student to practitioner. *PT Magazine.* 2001;9(11):24-26.

15. Lewis DK. Lessons from COURT [HPSO Web site]. HPSO Risk Advisor [serial online]. 2000;3(2):1-2. Available at: www.hpso.com. Accessed June 6, 2006.

## Chapter 3

# Documenting Patient/Client Management

*Mia Erickson, PT, EdD, CHT, ATC; Rebecca McKnight, PT, MS*

## Chapter Objectives

Upon completion of this chapter, the reader will be able to:

1. Describe components of the Patient/Client Management Model.
2. List requirements for documenting the initial visit with a patient.
3. Differentiate between the examination and evaluation according to the Patient/Client Management Model.
4. Realize the differing definitions for "evaluation."
5. Differentiate between subjective and objective data.
6. Realize the importance of documenting function and impairments.
7. List information that should be included in the evaluation, diagnosis, prognosis, and plan of care portions of the initial documentation.
8. Compare and contrast between interim (or treatment) notes and progress reports.
9. Differentiate between a short-term and a long-term goal.
10. Describe information to be included in a discharge note or summary.
11. Differentiate between discharge and discontinuation.

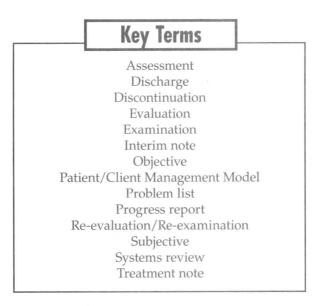

### Key Terms

Assessment
Discharge
Discontinuation
Evaluation
Examination
Interim note
Objective
Patient/Client Management Model
Problem list
Progress report
Re-evaluation/Re-examination
Subjective
Systems review
Treatment note

## Key Abbreviations

CMS
LTG
PTA
ROS
STG

# Documenting the Initial Patient Encounter

The initial patient encounter includes the initial examination and evaluation. The Patient/Client Management Model differentiates the examination from the evaluation in that the examination is the "process of ...gathering data about the patient/client,"[1(p43)] and evaluation is a process where the "physical therapist (PT) makes clinical judgments based on data gathered during the exam."[1(p43)] An additional point to be made here is that clinically, the terms *examination* and *evaluation* are often used synonymously. While *The Guide to Physical Therapist Practice* clearly differentiates between the terms and processes of examination and evaluation, clinically they are often collectively known as, "the initial evaluation." Additionally, the Centers for Medicare and Medicaid Services (CMS) recently defined *evaluation* as[2(p120)]:

a separately payable comprehensive service provided by a (physical therapist), that requires professional skills to make clinical judgments about conditions for which services are indicated based on objective measurements and subjective evaluations of patient performance and functional abilities. Evaluation is warranted, eg, for a new diagnosis or when a condition is treated in a new setting. These evaluative judgments are essential to development of the plan of care, including goals and the selection of interventions.

In order to be consistent with the *Guide* and the Patient/Client Management Model, throughout this text we will refer to *examination* as the process of collecting patient-related data, and the *evaluation* as the process of clinical decision making that occurs following the examination.

At the onset of the initial patient encounter, the PT goes through a process of collecting and recording data regarding the patient's current and prior medical conditions and functional status. As previously stated, the record of initial patient data provides baseline measurements to which future subjective and objective data can be compared. Comparisons to baseline measurements should be made throughout the episode of care to allow the PT to determine patient progress.[3]

While the examination, evaluation, and establishment of the plan of care are the sole responsibility of the physical therapist (PT), the PTA can assist the PT with the patient and with data collection.

Initial data collected are classified as subjective and objective. Subjective data are provided by the patient, a family member, or a caregiver, and include the history-taking portion of the examination. Data recorded during this phase include the physical therapy problem or reason for referral (Pr:), history of the present illness (HPI), mechanism of injury (MOI), date of injury (DOI) or onset date, prior medical history (PMH), information regarding the patient's lifestyle (L/S) such as living environment or situation, and the patient's goals for physical therapy. *The Guide to Physical Therapist Practice* also suggests collecting the following information (Appendix A)[1,4]:

- General patient demographics (age, sex, race, etc.)
- Social history/social support
- Employment/work history (job/school/play)
- Growth and developmental history
- Living environment
- General health (ie, health-related quality of life and previous medical history)
- Social/health habits (past and current)
- Family medical history
- Medical/surgical history
- Current condition(s)/chief complaints (c/c)
- Functional status/activity level (current and prior to the injury/illness)
- Medications
- Other clinical (or diagnostic) tests

Example 1 shows a sample patient record of subjective information collected during an initial examination.

After obtaining subjective information from the patient, family member, or caregiver, the PT will perform: 1) a systems review, and 2) the physical therapy tests and measures. These results provide objective data for the initial examination documentation. During a systems review, the PT assesses the

---

## Example 1. Sample of Subjective Documentation from Initial Encounter

**Patient name**: Becky Smith
**Date of service**: August 1, 2007
**Date of injury**: July 4, 2007

**Pr:** (R) humerus fracture; Referred to PT for shoulder and elbow PROM, sling on at all other times

**Subjective**: HPI: 67 y.o. white, right-hand dominant, female, 4 weeks s/p fall from chair while changing light bulb during which she sustained a (R) spiral humerus fracture. Immediately underwent ORIF and was placed in a sling. L/S: Pt. lives in two-story home with her husband. She has 2 grown children living nearby who can provide assistance. Pt. is a retired teacher who substitute teaches occasionally. Pt. plays recreational tennis and walks daily. She has been unable to perform normal ADLs including self-care, home management, driving, or exercising since the DOI Pt.'s Goal: Return to her normal active lifestyle. PMH: unremarkable. Pt. is a non-smoker and reports being in good health. She had a hysterectomy 15 years ago. C/C: Pain with motion of the (R) arm movements and difficulty performing self-care skills 2° to being unable to use her (R) arm. Reports using OTC ibuprofen for pain.

---

## Example 2. Sample of Systems Review Documentation from Initial Encounter

**Patient name**: Becky Smith
**Date of service**: August 1, 2007
**Date of injury**: July 4, 2007

**Pr**: (R) humerus fracture; Referred to PT for shoulder and elbow PROM, sling on at all other times

**Subjective**: HPI: 67 y.o. white, right-hand dominant, female, 4 weeks s/p fall from chair while changing light bulb which she sustained a (R) spiral humerus fracture. Immediately underwent ORIF and was placed in a sling. L/S: Pt. lives in two-story home with her husband. She has 2 grown children living near by who can provide assistance. Pt. is a retired teacher who substitute teaches occasionally. Pt. plays recreational tennis and walks daily. She has been unable to perform normal ADLs including self-care, home management, drive, or exercise since the DOI Pt.'s Goal: to return to her normal active lifestyle. PMH: Unremarkable. Pt. is a non-smoker and reports being in good health. She had a hysterectomy 15 years ago. C/C: Pain with motion of the (R) arm movements and difficulty performing self-care skills 2° to being unable to use her (R) arm. Reports using OTC ibuprofen for pain.

**ROS**: Cardiopulmonary system: HR: 88, BP: 128/88, RR: 10. Integumentary system: Incision healed, immature scar present along posterior humerus. Musculoskeletal system: Pt. is 5' 7" and 155#. (R) UE held at her side in a sling, decreased (R) shoulder and elbow AROM, (R) AROM wrist and hand is WNL. All (L) UE and cervical AROM is WNL. Neuromuscular system: She ambulated (I) into the clinic without difficulty. Gross sensation to light touch (B) is intact. Communicates without difficulty.

---

patient's overall condition by grossly screening the cardiovascular/pulmonary (ie, heart rate, blood pressure, respiratory rate), integumentary, musculoskeletal, and neuromuscular systems. The PT also screens the patient's cognitive and communication abilities during the systems review (Appendix A) (Example 2).[1]

Based upon information gleaned during the systems review, the PT selects and performs more specific tests and measures to further examine the patient's status. These more specific tests and measures allow the PT to accurately pinpoint and measure physical therapy impairments, functional deficits, and limitations in life roles and tasks. These measurements are crucial for establishing the physical therapy diagnosis, prognosis, and plan of care. A list of specific tests and measures used by the PT during the initial examination can be found in *The Guide to Physical Therapist Practice*[1] and in the *Guidelines for Physical Therapy Documentation of Patient/Client Management* (Appendix A).[4]

Impairments in range of motion (ROM), strength, sensation, circulation, limb circumference, and balance are often measured in a PT's examination

## Example 3. Sample of Tests and Measures (Impairments) Documentation from Initial Encounter

**Patient name**: Becky Smith

**Date of service**: August 1, 2007

**Date of injury**: July 4, 2007

**Pr:** (R) humerus fracture; Referred to PT for shoulder and elbow PROM, sling on at all other times

**Subjective**: HPI: 67 y.o. white, right-hand dominant, female, 4 weeks s/p fall from chair while changing light bulb which she sustained a (R) spiral humerus fracture. Immediately underwent ORIF and was placed in a sling. L/S: Pt. lives in two-story home with her husband. She has 2 grown children living near by who can provide assistance. Pt. is a retired teacher who substitute teaches occasionally. Pt. plays recreational tennis and walks daily. She has been unable to perform normal ADLs including self-care, home management, drive, or exercise since the DOI Pt.'s Goal: to return to her normal active lifestyle. PMH: Unremarkable. Pt. is a non-smoker and reports being in good health. She had a hysterectomy 15 years ago. C/C: Pain with motion of the (R) arm movements and difficulty performing self-care skills 2° to being unable to use her (R) arm. Reports using OTC ibuprofen for pain.

**ROS**: Cardiopulmonary system: HR: 88, BP: 128/88, RR: 10. Integumentary system: Incision healed Musculoskeletal system: Pt. is 5' 7" and 155#. (R) UE held at her side in a sling, decreased (R) shoulder and elbow ROM, (R) AROM wrist and hand is WNL. All (L) UE and cervical AROM is WNL. Neuromuscular system: She ambulated (I) into the clinic without difficulty. Gross sensation to light touch (B) is intact. Communicates without difficulty.

**Tests and measures**: Capillary refill: intact Integumentary integrity: immature adhered scar present along posterior humerus, dry, hypersensitive to touch, raised ~1-2 mm Strength: (L) UE 5/5; (R) UE N/A this visit 2° to surgery Pain rating: at rest 2/10, at worst 6/10 PROM: (R) shoulder: flexion 95° abduction 90° ER 35° IR 50°; elbow: -10/100°; (L) shoulder: flexion 160° abduction 160° ER 90° IR 70°; elbow 0/140°

---

(Example 3). However, with the shifting focus from impairment toward function and disability, the use of standardized functional performance instruments has become more popular. Examining and documenting functional status provides more specific, contextual information regarding the impact of the pathologies and impairments on the patient's life roles and normal activities (Example 4). We know from Chapter 1 that mere presence of impairment does not always correlate to a functional problem. Furthermore, individuals reviewing medical records often deem the patient's functional status as being more meaningful than documentation of impairments alone.

Functional measures can be performance-based, ie, requiring the patient to perform a set of functional tasks. An example of a performance-based assessment is the Functional Independence Measure (FIM). Functional assessments can also be "self-report," where the patient completes a questionnaire rating his or her overall performance on a predetermined set of functional tasks. An example of a patient self-reported functional measure is the Oswestry Low Back Pain Disability Questionnaire, often used to assess the functional status of patients with back pain. Other examples of self-reported pain and/or disability questionnaires include the Short-Form 36 Health Survey

(SF-36), the Patient-Rated Wrist Evaluation (PRWE), and the Neck Disability Index (NDI).

The PT uses the information and data gathered during the examination process to make a clinical judgment about the patient's condition. Again, according to the Patient/Client Management Model, this clinical judgment is known as the evaluation.[1] You may also hear this process referred to as the impression or assessment. According to the Patient/Client Management Model, the evaluation is actually a thought process, or clinical problem-solving process, where the PT considers all data gathered to establish the patient's plan of care.[1,4] The evaluation process guides the PT in determining and documenting the physical therapy diagnosis, the patient's prognosis, and the plan of care. Information documented during the evaluation, diagnosis, prognosis, and plan of care includes[4,5]:

1. A brief summary of the patient
   - Synthesizing the exam findings and correlating impairments to functional deficits and limitations in life roles and tasks
   - An explanation of the need for skilled services

## Example 4. Sample of Tests and Measures (Function) Documentation from Initial Encounter

**Patient name**: Becky Smith

**Date of service**: August 1, 2007

**Date of injury**: July 4, 2007

**Pr**: (R) humerus fracture; Referred to PT for shoulder and elbow PROM, sling on at all other times

**Subjective**: HPI: 67 y.o. white, right-hand dominant, female, 4 weeks s/p fall from chair while changing light bulb which she sustained a (R) spiral humerus fracture. Immediately underwent ORIF and was placed in a sling. L/S: Pt. lives in two-story home with her husband. She has 2 grown children living near by who can provide assistance. Pt. is a retired teacher who substitute teaches occasionally. Pt. plays recreational tennis and walks daily. She has been unable to perform normal ADLs including self-care, home management, drive, or exercise since the DOI Pt.'s Goal: to return to her normal active lifestyle. PMH: Unremarkable. Pt. is a non-smoker and reports being in good health. She had a hysterectomy 15 years ago. C/C: Pain with motion of the (R) arm movements and difficulty performing self-care skills 2° to being unable to use her (R) arm. Reports using OTC ibuprofen for pain.

**ROS**: Cardiopulmonary system: HR: 88, BP: 128/88, RR: 10. Integumentary system: Incision healed Musculoskeletal system: Pt. is 5' 7" and 155#. (R) UE held at her side in a sling, decreased (R) shoulder and elbow ROM, (R) AROM wrist and hand is WNL. All (L) UE and cervical AROM is WNL. Neuromuscular system: She ambulated (I) into the clinic without difficulty. Gross sensation to light touch (B) is intact. Communicates without difficulty.

**Tests and measures**: Capillary refill: intact Integumentary integrity: immature adhered scar present along posterior humerus, dry, hypersensitive to touch, raised ~1-2 mm Strength: (L) UE 5/5; (R) UE N/A this visit 2° to surgery Pain rating: at rest 2/10, at worst 6/10 PROM: (R) shoulder: flexion 95° abduction 90° ER 35° IR 50°; elbow: -10/100°; (L) shoulder: flexion 160° abduction 160° ER 90° IR 70°; elbow 0/140°

**Functional assessment**: DASH questionnaire score 84/100, see attached; Requires assistance with ADLs including hygiene, dressing, and bathing; unable to complete home management tasks, drive, work, or participate in normal recreational activities, i.e., tennis, walking program

---

2. Physical therapy diagnosis

- The physical therapy diagnosis (can be ICD- 9 or a practice pattern from *The Guide to Physical Therapist Practice*) (Appendix D)

- The patient's physical therapy problems (impairments, functional deficits, limitations in normal life roles and tasks) written in a format often called *the problem list*

3. Patient Prognosis

- Potential for improvement, or rehabilitation potential

- Factors that may influence treatment and/ or progress (medical, cognitive, psychological, social, economic, etc.). These are known as co-morbidities, complexities, or complicating factors

- Specific, objective, measurable goals providing a predicted level of improvement with a set time frame for achievement. Goals serve as a PT's "measuring stick" for monitoring patient progress and determining the effec-

tiveness of the treatment and plan of care. These are written as discharge or outcome goals. These may also be referred to as long-term goals (LTGs). Short-term goals (STGs) may also be added. A STG is a stepping stone toward the final discharge goals (Note: occasionally, goals are considered part of the plan of care in addition to the prognosis). Short-term goals are written in a manner consistent with the discharge/outcome goal on which it is based. See the following example:

*Example*:

Discharge goal 1: The patient will be an independent ambulator without an assistive device in 8 weeks.

A corresponding initial STG could be:

STG 1-A: The patient will be able to ambulate 200' with a straight cane on level surfaces in 2 weeks.

4. Plan of care
   - The suggested interventions:

   A general statement or list of specific interventions to be used including:

   1. coordination/communication with other disciplines, or individuals involved in the patient's care, or referrals to other providers
   2. patient education to be provided
   3. procedural or therapeutic interventions

   - The expected frequency, amount, and duration of services

*Frequency*: Number of times per week the patient will be treated, eg, 2-3x/wk

*Amount*: Number of times per day the patient will be treated. If no amount is specified then one time per day is often assumed, eg, 5x/wk bid

*Duration*: Length of the entire episode of care, or time to discharge. This is usually specified in weeks or months, eg, 3x/wk x 8 wks

   - The ultimate discharge plan (eg, return to work, return to prior level of function, discharge to long-term care facility, discharge to inpatient rehabilitation facility). This may also be included in the goals.

Example 5 provides completed examination and evaluative documentation from an initial encounter. A summary of all information found in the initial documentation for each element of Patient/Client Management can be found in Table 3-1. These general guidelines can be applied to an inpatient or outpatient setting and they also satisfy documentation requirements for the outpatient initial plan of care set forth by CMS. A template for initial documentation can also be found in Appendix C.

# Documenting Subsequent Encounters

## Interim Notes

As the physical therapy interventions are initiated, the patient's progress toward the established goals is monitored and documented. This includes collecting and recording similar subjective and objective data that were documented during the initial encounter. Subsequent patient encounters, visits, or treatment sessions are documented in interim notes. *Interim notes* are also called treatment encounter notes, daily notes, or progress notes. These interim notes are written to maintain ongoing records of subjective and objective data; specific intervention(s) provided;

results of the intervention(s); the patient's response(s) to the interventions in terms of impairments, function, and disability; changes (or need for changes) in the plan of care; need for referral to another practitioner; and plans for subsequent treatment/intervention.[4] These interim notes also serve as a record of services provided to patients to support what was billed, or charged to the patient on a given date.

New regulations from CMS recently differentiated between two types of interim notes for physical therapy delivered to Medicare beneficiaries in an outpatient setting. These are Treatment Encounter Notes and Progress Reports. The Treatment Encounter Note "is not required to document medical necessity or appropriateness of the ongoing therapy services."[2(p151)] At *minimum*, the Treatment Encounter Note includes[2]:

- Date of treatment
- Identification of each procedure/modality provided and billed, for both timed and untimed codes (see Chapter 11), in language that can be compared with the billing on the claim to verify correct coding
- Total timed code treatment minutes
- Total treatment time in minutes (excluding time for services *not* billable)
- Signature and professional designation of the qualified professional who furnished or supervised the services and a list of persons who contributed (see Appendix C for a template of a Treatment Encounter Note).

According to CMS, the Treatment Encounter Note is different from the Progress Report in that "the Progress Report provides justification for the medical necessity of treatment."[2(p146)] The current requirement is that a Progress Report is written for Medicare beneficiaries being treated in an outpatient setting at least once every 10 treatment days or at least once a month (whichever is less). Requirements for Progress Reports include:[2(p149-150)]

- Dates of treatment interval (current date and date of last Progress Report or initial exam/evaluation)
- Date the report is written if different from above
- Signature and professional designation of the PT who wrote the report
- Objective report of the patient's relevant subjective comments
- Objective measurements including a description of changes in status. These should be related to current treatment goals
- Documentation of any progress toward *or* changes in goals

## Example 5. Sample of Evaluation, Prognosis, Diagnosis, and Plan of Care Documentation from Initial Encounter

**Patient Name**: Becky Smith

**Date of service:** August 1, 2007

**Date of injury**: July 4, 2007

**Pr**: (R) humerus fracture; Referred to PT for shoulder and elbow PROM, sling on at all other times; next MD visit 2 weeks

**Subjective**: <u>HPI</u>: 67 y.o. white, right-hand dominant, female, 4 weeks s/p fall from chair while changing light bulb which she sustained a (R) spiral humerus fracture. Immediately underwent ORIF and was placed in a sling. <u>L/S</u>: Pt. lives in two-story home with her husband. She has 2 grown children living near by who can provide assistance. Pt. is a retired teacher who substitute teaches occasionally. Pt. plays recreational tennis and walks daily. She has been unable to perform normal ADLs including self-care, home management, drive, or exercise since the DOI <u>Pt.'s Goal</u>: to return to her normal active lifestyle. <u>PMH</u>: Unremarkable. Pt. is a non-smoker and reports being in good health. She had a hysterectomy 15 years ago. <u>C/C</u>: Pain with motion of the (R) arm movements and difficulty performing self-care skills 2° to being unable to use her (R) arm. Reports using OTC ibuprofen for pain.

**ROS**: <u>Cardiopulmonary system</u>: HR: 88, BP: 128/88, RR: 10. <u>Integumentary system</u>: Incision healed <u>Musculoskeletal system</u>: Pt. is 5' 7" and 155#. (R) UE held at her side in a sling, decreased (R) shoulder and elbow ROM, (R) AROM wrist and hand is WNL. All (L) UE and cervical AROM is WNL. <u>Neuromuscular system</u>: She ambulated (I) into the clinic without difficulty. Gross sensation to light touch (B) is intact. Communicates without difficulty.

**Tests and measures**: <u>Capillary refill</u>: intact Integumentary integrity: immature adhered scar present along posterior humerus, dry, hypersensitive to touch, raised ~1-2 mm Strength: (L) UE 5/5; (R) UE N/A this visit 2° to surgery <u>Pain rating</u>: at rest 2/10, at worst 6/10 <u>PROM</u>: (R) shoulder: flexion 95° abduction 90° ER 35° IR 50°; elbow: -10/100°; (L) shoulder: flexion 160° abduction 160° ER 90° IR 70°; elbow 0/140°

**Functional assessment**: DASH questionnaire score 84/100, see attached; Requires assistance with ADLs including hygiene, dressing, and bathing; unable to complete home management tasks, drive, work, or participate in normal recreational activities, i.e., tennis, walking program

**Evaluation and Plan**: Pt. is 4 weeks s/p ORIF humerus (ICD-9 code: 812) referred for shoulder and elbow PROM to dominant extremity; ROM limitations in place by surgeon to protect healing fracture causing inability to use extremity for ADLs, home tasks or driving. Skilled services needed for mobilizing (R) shoulder and elbow while protecting healing fracture. <u>PT Problems</u>: Impairments: 1) decreased ROM (R) UE, 2) decreased strength (R) UE; 3) adhered scar; 4) pain <u>Function</u>: 1) DASH score 84/100 indicating 84% disability; 2) requiring assistance with ADLs; 3) unable to perform normal life roles including home management tasks, driving, work activities, and recreational activities <u>PT Diagnosis</u>: Practice Pattern 4G. <u>Prognosis</u>: Pt. has good social support and is motivated, demonstrating good potential to return to normal lifestyle and to meet established goals.

<u>Discharge Goals</u> (to be met in 8 weeks):

1) AROM (R) UE 90-100% of (L)

2) Strength (R) 4 to 4+/5

3) Non-adhered, mobile scar

4) Pain 0/10

5) DASH score < 25%

6) Independent in all ADLs

*(continued)*

## Example 5. Sample of Evaluation, Prognosis, Diagnosis, and Plan of Care Documentation from Initial Encounter, Continued

7) Independent in home management

8) Return to driving without limitations

9) Return to work without limitations

10) Return to mild recreational activities in 8 weeks with anticipated full return in 12 weeks

<u>Interventions</u>: Pt. will be treated on outpatient basis 2-3x per week for 8 weeks using therapeutic exercises and modalities to improve ROM, pain, and scar formation. Pt. will also be instructed in a home exercise program. Progressing pt. to functional activities and strength when allowed by surgeon.

Table 3-1

## Documentation of the Patient's Initial Encounter With the Physical Therapist

| Component of Patient/Client Management | Includes: | Source of information: | What to record: |
|---|---|---|---|
| Examination | 1) History | Patient/Family/Caregiver interview | • Subjective data |
| | 2) Systems review: Cardiovascular System Integumentary System Musculoskeletal System Neuromuscular System Cognitive/Communicative ability | Medical record/chart Gross examination of body systems | • Objective data—Results of systems review and tests and measures |
| | 3) Tests and measures | Specific physical therapy tests and measures (eg, range of motion, strength, etc.) | |
| Evaluation | Clinical judgment, problem-solving process, PT diagnosis and prognosis, and established plan of care | Results of the examination and the clinician's problem-solving skills/clinical judgment | •Brief summary of the patient, synthesizing exam findings, including relationship between impairments and function<br>• PT problems and need for skilled services<br>•Factors influencing treatment (eg, co-morbidities)<br>•PT diagnosis (can use ICD-9 or a practice pattern from *The Guide to Physical Therapist Practice*)<br>• Rehab potential<br>• Physical therapy goals<br>• Planned interventions including frequency, duration, and amount of treatment<br>• Discharge plans |

(Reference: American Physical Therapy Association. Defensible documentation. Available at: http://www.apta.org/AM/Template.cfm?Section=Home&NAVMENUID=2505&CONTENTID=37071&DIRECTLISTCOMBOIND=D&TEMPLATE=/MembersOnly.cfm. Accessed July 30, 2007.)

- Document if a STG has been met and record new STGs with reference to the corresponding discharge/outcome goal:

*Example*:
Discharge goal 1: The patient will be an independent community ambulator without an assistive device in 8 weeks.

STG 1-A: The patient will be able to ambulate 200' with a straight cane on level surfaces in 2 weeks (Goal Met)

New STG 1-B: The patient will ambulate 500' without an assistive device on level surfaces in 2 weeks.

- Document changes to existing discharge/outcome goals

*Example*:
Discharge goal 2 in current plan deleted.
- An overall assessment of progress, or lack thereof
- Plans and justification for continuing treatment given that:
  –The patient's condition has the potential to improve

  –Maximum improvement is yet to be attained

  –The expectation is that maximum improvement will occur within a reasonable and generally predictable amount of time

Again, this differentiation between Treatment Encounter Notes and Progress Reports is specific for documentation for Medicare beneficiaries receiving treatment in an outpatient setting. However, specific payers' regulations are updated or changed frequently, so as a practicing clinician, you will need to continually stay up-to-date in documentation requirements. One way to stay current with the CMS regulations is to check periodically on the CMS web site (www.cms.gov). At the time of writing this text, the requirements were found in the Medicare Benefit Policy Manual, Internet Only Manuals, Chapter 15, Section 220. See Appendix C for a template of a progress report.

## Timing Interim Notes

In some physical therapy settings such as outpatient clinics, acute care hospitals, and home health, interim notes are written for each visit or encounter the PT or PTA has with a patient. However, in other settings, like acute rehabilitation and skilled nursing facilities, these interim notes are often written on a weekly basis, summarizing the patient's status and progress toward goals. Federal rules or regulations, state laws, and facility policies dictate the frequency of documentation in various settings.

## Assessments and Re-Evaluations

Throughout the episode of care, PTs and PTAs maintain a record of changes in the patient's status. Data collection can be carried out through regular assessments or through more formal re-evaluations. An assessment includes gathering subjective and objective data to determine whether the patient is making progress toward his or her stated goals. These regular assessments are expected by third-party payers, and usually occur on a weekly basis. Regular assessments are documented in interim, encounter, or progress reports.

These ongoing assessments are different from formal re-evaluations. In a Medicare transmittal, re-evaluation was defined as[2]:

> additional objective information not included in other documentation...separately payable and indicated during an episode of care when the professional assessment indicates a significant improvement, decline, or change in condition or functional status that was not anticipated.

Re-evaluations are more formal, thorough, complete records of the patient's status, including tests and measures from the initial encounter, any additional tests and measures, and record of new developments or problems the patient may be having. In addition, the re-evaluation includes specific progress (or lack thereof) toward goals stated on the plan of care. Re-evaluations should occur when there are significant changes in the patient's status or within a required time frame dictated by state or federal law or facility policy.

After considering the assessment or re-evaluation findings, the PT again uses his or her clinical judgment to determine whether the current plan of care should be continued or changed. Changing the plan of care involves changing the patient's goals; interventions; frequency, amount, or duration of services; or ultimate discharge plan. Changes to the plan of care require justification, and this can be done by calling the reader's attention to the subjective or objective data collected that warrants the change.

## Discharge

*The Guide to Physical Therapist Practice* defines discharge as ending services provided in a single episode of care, when goals and outcomes have been achieved.[1] When the patient is being discharged from physical therapy services, the patient's subjective and objective data are provided in a discharge note or summary to outline his or her final status. Any data recorded in a discharge note must be compared to data collected from the initial encounter so that the medical record reflects both subjective and objective changes in the patient's status achieved throughout the episode of care. In the discharge summary, the PT documents the patient's progress toward the established goals, plans for continuing care elsewhere, or the patient's final outcome.[4]

*The Guide to Physical Therapist Practice* differentiates discharge from discontinuation.[1] *Discontinuation* is defined as the process of ending services provided in an episode of care when the patient: 1) declines further intervention; 2) is unable to participate, as in cases when there is a significant change in the medical condition or there is a change in financial or psychosocial resources allowing the patient to continue; or 3) will no longer benefit. Nevertheless, clinically, the term *discharge* is most often used to denote ending the episode of care regardless of the reason.

# The Physical Therapist Assistant and Interim Notes

The state's physical therapy practice act determines what the PTA can legally document. In many cases, however, the PTA can write subjective and objective data. Additionally, the PTA can add comments as to changes in objective data from previous visits. For example:

A PTA has been working with Mr. Smith for the last three treatments for gait training after a total knee arthroplasty. On day 1 of treatment, the patient ambulated 50 feet with minimal assist for balance. On treatment day 3, the patient ambulated 150 feet requiring close supervision.

The PTA can call attention to these specific changes in status, documenting:

Ambulation improved from 50' with minimal assist to 150' with supervision.

Nevertheless, it is the sole responsibility of the PT to write the evaluative portions of the initial documentation, assessments, re-evaluations, and discharge notes. This includes the prognosis, diagnosis, and plan of care as well as provision of any changes within or to the plan of care.

---

# Review Questions

1. Differentiate the *examination* process from the *evaluation* process according to the Patient/Client Management Model.

2. In a clinical setting *and* according to CMS, examination and evaluation are collectively referred to as _____.

3. Subjective data are taken from_____.

4. List five examples of subjective data.

5. Following collection of subjective data (history-taking), the PT should perform: _____ and _____.

6. The results of a. and b. above are considered _____ data.

7. During the examination, the PT measures impairment *and* _____.

8. Give two reasons for documenting impairment *and* function.

9. The evaluation process guides the PT in determining and documenting the _____, _____, and _____.

10. The "summary" of the patient provided in the evaluative portion of the note should serve to link _____ and _____.

11. Factors such as a secondary medical diagnosis that adversely influence treatment are known as _____.

12. Goals written on the initial documentation are _____, or _____ goals.

13. Differentiate between a Treatment Encounter Note and a Progress Note, according to CMS.

14. What information must be included in the progress note that is not required to be in the treatment encounter note.

15. How are short-term goals related to outcome or discharge goals?

16. Differentiate between regular assessments and re-evaluations.

17. In what settings are progress notes written on a weekly basis, rather than for each encounter?

18. A PT can bill separately for a _____, as opposed to a regular assessment, which is expected and not separately billable.

19. List five things found in a discharge summary.

20. How does *The Guide to Physical Therapist Practice* differentiate *discharge* from *discontinuation*?

## Application Exercises

I. Look through *The Guide to PT Practice* and identify 10 common tests and measures used by PTs. Differentiate those that measure impairments from those that measure function.

II.  Match the appropriate short-term goal for the following outcome goals.

| Outcome Goal: | Short-term Goals (STGs) |
|---|---|
| _____1. The patient will ambulate with prosthesis 500' without assistive device on varied terrain. | A. The patient will manage his wheelchair on a variety of surfaces 250' with minimal verbal cueing. |
| _____2. The patient will transfer independently to and from all surfaces with supervision. | B. The patient will transfer to and from the right side independently and to and from the left side with minimal assist. |
| _____3. The patient will manage his wheelchair independently for 500' in an open environment independently to allow independent community mobility. | C. The patient will ambulate 75' with a standard walker and the prosthesis with minimal assist for balance and weight shifting. |
| _____4. The patient will ambulate 150' with prosthesis and quad cane independently on level surfaces. | D. The patient will propel his wheelchair on level surfaces 50 to 75' with verbal cues. |
| _____5. The patient will manage his wheelchair 100' on level surfaces and small inclines independently. | E. The patient will ambulate 250' with prosthesis and quad cane on level surfaces and small inclines with supervision and verbal cues. |

III.  Look at the initial examination and evaluation note on the following page. Identify:
 1. Three pieces of subjective information
 2. Three pieces of objective data
 3. The patient summary
 4. The physical therapy diagnosis
 5. The patient's problems
 6. An explanation of the need for skilled services
 7. Co-morbidities
 8. Referral to another provider
 9. Outcome goals
 10. List of interventions
 11. Frequency, amount, and duration of services
 12. Ultimate plan for discharge

*This patient was admitted to an inpatient rehabilitation unit 4 days after transtibial amputation.*

Date: January 15, 2004

**Pr**: 72-year-old male 4 days s/p (R) transtibial amputation
**S**: HPI: Long history of chronic wounds on the (R) foot; recently developed osteomyelitis and gangrene and underwent short transtibial (BK) amputation. C/C: Phantom pain from the (L) foot, poor mobility, and decreased endurance. L/S: Pt. is retired coal miner. Lives alone in single-level house, with 2 steps at the entrance. Has never used an assistive device. Has been independent with all ADLs and IADLs prior to admission. PMH: NIDDM, COPD, PVD, and HTN. Pt. is a non-smoker and non-drinker, although smoked 1 pack per day for 30 years. Quit when he was 50 y.o. Has one son living about 2 hours away who can assist on the weekends. Pt's Goals: Return to independent, active L/S, including driving. Wants to obtain a prosthetic device.
**O**: ROS: CP System: HR 92 bpm, BP 135/88, RR 12 Integumentary System: sutures present along anterior aspect of the distal tibia; Musculoskeletal System: Height 6′ 2″ Weight 225# AROM (B) UEs is WNL, (L) LE AROM is WNL, (R) LE AROM is decreased 2° to surgery (see specific ROM measurements below) Neuromuscular system: Decreased sensation to light touch around the scar and on the (L) foot. Communication: Pt. communicates goals and needs without difficulty.
Tests and measures:
Capillary refill: (L) foot is intact Incision: 5″ horizontal incision, minimal red bloody drainage, no tension, complete closure, no s/s of infection AROM: (R) hip flexion 90°, extension 0°, abduction 40°, adduction 10°, knee flexion 60°, knee extension -10°. PROM: (R) hip flexion 95°, knee extension -5°, knee flexion 65°. Strength: (B) UEs and (L) LE are 4/5 throughout; (R) LE not assessed 2° to surgery. Pulses: Popliteal artery 2+ (B). Residual limb length: 2″ from tibial tuberosity.

| Edema: | (R) | (L) |
|---|---|---|
| Knee joint | 22 cm | 20 cm |
| 2″ below | 22.5 cm | 19 cm |

Balance: Not impaired when standing in // bars. Endurance: unable to ambulate more than 25′ without shortness of breath. Bed Mobility: independent rolling and scooting. Transfers: supine → sit with minimal assist x 1; sit → stand with minimal assist x 1; toilet transfers performed with minimal assist x 1. Gait: Ambulated 10′ x 1 in // bars with contact guard assist x 1 and 25′ with standard walker with minimal assist x 1. Balance impaired when ambulating with walker. Wheelchair management: Requires maximal assist for wheelchair management; propels ~ 20′ on level surfaces and then requires a rest break. Ther Ex: 20 minutes of exercises including hip AROM: flexion, extension, abduction, and adduction; knee flexion and extension; hamstring stretching, and towel propping.
**A**: 72 y.o. male 4 days s/p (R) transtibial amputation with decreased ROM, strength, and balance resulting in impaired mobility including transfers and functional ambulation. PT diagnosis: Impaired motor function, muscle performance, range of motion, gait, locomotion, and balance associated with amputation. Patient requiring skilled services for improving functional mobility including gait and transfer training with assistive devices 2° to amputation. Also required for preparing residual limb for prosthesis.
Problem List:
Impairments:
      1) decreased ROM (R) LE
      2) decreased strength (R) LE
      3) decreased sensation
      4) edema
      5) incision present
      6) impaired balance with walker
      7) phantom pain
      8) impaired endurance

Functional Limitations:
      1) decreased independence with ambulation
      2) decreased independence with transfers
      3) unable to drive
      4) unable to perform necessary IADLs (grocery shopping, going to bank, etc)
      5) unable to participate in active L/S using a prosthetic device

Prognosis is good for established goals and outcomes although complexities such as COPD, PVD, HTN, impaired endurance and decreased sensation on the (L) LE may slow progress.

Discharge Goals: After 8 weeks pt. will:
1. Demonstrate full A/PROM in the (R) LE with no contractures—necessary for normal prosthetic ambulation
2. (R) LE strength 4/5 also to allow normal prosthetic ambulation
3. Be independent with skin care and monitoring skin with use of prosthesis on the (L) LE
4. Ambulate 200′ with walker with prosthesis and least restrictive assistive device (I)
5. Transfer in/out of bed and sit → stand of bed independently
6. Participate in a community outing with only minimal assist x 1
7. Obtain driving assessment
8. Return home independently and obtain appropriate home modifications and equipment

**P**: See pt. for 1 hour bid for ~ 8 weeks to work on achieving the above goals through active and passive exercise, strengthening, endurance training, gait and transfer training, pain modulation, balance, and pt. education. Pt. will also require occupational therapy assessment and consultation with prosthetist. The patient is motivated and agrees with the above plan.

# References

1. American Physical Therapy Association. *The Guide to Physical Therapist Practice*. Alexandria, VA: APTA; 2001.
2. Centers for Medicare and Medicaid Services. Medicare Benefit Policy Manual. Centers for Medicare and Medicaid Services Web site; Internet-Only Manuals: 2006. Publication No. 100-02, Ch. 15-Section 220.
3. Hebert LA. Basics of Medicare documentation for physical therapy. *Clinical Management in Physical Therapy*. 1981;1(3):13-4.
4. American Physical Therapy Association. Guidelines: Physical Therapy Documentation of Patient/Client Management. Available at: http://www.apta.org/AM/Template.cfm?Section=Policies_and_Bylaws&TEMPLATE=/CM/ContentDisplay.cfm&CONTENTID=31688. Accessed July 7, 2007.
5. American Physical Therapy Association. Defensible documentation. Available at: http://www.apta.org/AM/Template.cfm?Section=Home&NAVMENUID=2505&CONTENTID=37071&DIRECTLISTCOMBOIND=D&TEMPLATE=/MembersOnly.cfm. Accessed July 30, 2007.

## Chapter 4

# Documentation Formats

*Mia Erickson, PT, EdD, CHT, ATC*

## Chapter Objectives

Upon completion of this chapter, the reader will be able to:

1. Compare and contrast narrative notes, SOAP notes, problem-oriented medical records (POMR), and functional outcomes reports (FOR).
2. Differentiate between information found in the S, O, A, and P portions of a SOAP note.
3. Explain the rationale for blending SOAP and FOR.
4. Organize patient information using the different documentation formats.

### Key Terms

Functional outcome report
Narrative notes
Problem-oriented medical record
SOAP note

### Key Abbreviations

A:
FOR
O:
P:
POMR
Pr:
S:

# Documentation Formats

Documentation in physical therapy practice can take on a variety of formats, and the format you use will depend on the type of patients being treated, the practice setting, state laws and practice acts, reimbursement requirements, and the type of patient encounter. Different documentation formats include: narrative reports, problem-oriented medical records (POMR), SOAP, and functional outcomes reporting (FOR). A brief discussion of each of these formats is provided below.

## Narrative Notes

In narrative documentation, the clinician describes the patient encounter with pertinent information provided in paragraph format. The narrative format can be used when documenting initial patient encounters (Example 1A), interim notes (Example 1B), re-evaluations or reassessments (Example 1C), and discharge summaries (Example 1D). Besides typical patient care documentation, there are other times when the narrative format is the most appropriate to use. These include describing a sequence of events, brief interactions with patients, conversations with other health care providers, or any other situation that requires a detailed explanation and no other documentation formats are appropriate (Example 1E). In these instances, you can simply describe the situation in a brief narrative note. Narrative notes are sometimes the easiest to use when you just need to describe the details of a situation and you are trying to paint a vivid description of what happened.

Authors have identified several problems with the narrative record. First, due to the lack of structure, the writer is prone to omit details that could potentially be very important. The lack of structure combined with a high degree of variability among clinicians writing in this format, make narrative notes difficult to read and locate necessary information.[1] For example, following the clinician's problem-solving process can be difficult in narrative reports.[2] Additionally, it would be very time-consuming for a case manager to sort through a chart filled with unstructured narrative entries to locate information regarding the patient's ability to transfer. For these reasons, more structured documentation formats have emerged.

Quinn and Gordon[1] recommended developing an outline of necessary information to include so that important details about the patient or the treatment session are not omitted. Headings can also be used to denote different sections or different types of data. The use of headings gives the narrative note structure, makes the narrative note more readable, and allows someone to find information in the note more quickly. Headings often used are shown in Table 4-1.

## Problem-Oriented Medical Record

The Problem-Oriented Medical Record (POMR) was developed by Lawrence Weed in the 1960s. Weed[2] indicated that narrative documentation was confusing and unorganized, making it difficult to use. The POMR, used mainly by medical students and physicians at the time, organizes patient information and treatment according to the patient's problems. The first page of the medical record includes the patient-problem list, and this serves as the "Table of Contents" for the remainder of the medical record (Example 2A). After documentation of the initial encounter, subsequent entries, or interim notes, provide subjective and objective clinical data, an overall impression (Abbreviated as "Imp:"), treatment or therapy (Abbreviated as "Tx:" or "Rx:"), and a future plan for each problem (Example 2B). Using this format, the reader can quickly identify the care provided and future plans for each of the patient's problems.

Major advantages of POMR have been reported.[3-7] The POMR:

- Provides organization and structure to the medical information

- Includes a comprehensive list of the patient's problems

- Discusses each of the patient's problems and care provided separately

- Provides a specific plan for managing each of the patient's problems (ie, treatment is problem-oriented)

| Documentation Formats | Description |
| --- | --- |
| • Narrative | Information provided in paragraph format |
| • Problem-oriented medical record | Organized according to patient problems |
| • SOAP | Organized according to subjective, objective, assessment, and plan |
| • Functional outcomes report | Organized according to patient problems |
| • Blend | Integrates functional outcomes reporting into SOAP format |

## Example 1A. Initial Examination and Evaluation—Narrative Format

*PT Examination and Evaluation*

**Patient**: John Smith
**Date of Service**: January 3, 2006

Mr. Smith is a 35 y.o. male referred to PT by Dr. Jones for pain in the (L) lateral elbow. Medical diagnosis is (L) lateral epicondylitis. Pt. reports developing pain after spending the weekend painting his house 3 months ago. The pt. reports using ice and taking meds (OTC ibuprofen) initially but this didn't help. Saw his physician for a yearly physical and mentioned the elbow pain. His MD suggested "trying a few weeks of PT." Chief complaint at this time is pain (6/10 at worst and 2/10 at best) that increases with heavy grip, computer use, and using hand tools. Denies temperature changes and numbness. Has not had any x-rays or imaging procedures. Pt. denies hx of a similar problem and prior elbow pain. Reports overall health is good with no relevant medical or surgical history. Pt. lives alone and works as an accountant. Reports primary functional deficits include painful work-related activities, home management tasks, and recreational activities such as mountain biking and kayaking. Global functional rating is 85% out of 100. The pt.'s goals for therapy include pain reduction allowing improvement in functional tasks and prevention of recurrence. Review of systems revealed BP: 120/84, HR: 78 bpm, and RR: 12. Neurological and integumentary systems are not impaired. No impairments in cognitive or communicative status. Musculoskeletal system shows palpable point tenderness on the (L) lateral epicondyle and wrist extensor origin. AROM of (R) UE is WNL (elbow 0/145°); (L) shoulder, wrist, and hand are WNL, elbow is –10/140°; c/o pain at end range elbow flexion, extension, and wrist extension; cervical A/PROM also WNL and pain free. PROM of the (L) elbow is 0/145 with normal end feel but c/o pain. MMT indicates 5/5 strength throughout (B) UE except (L) wrist extension and supination are 4/5 with pain. All provocation tests for (L) elbow are unremarkable except a (+) tennis elbow test. Pain free grip strength (R) 100, 110, 108#; (L) 65, 60, 55# with pain. (-) edema compared bil. Neurovascular structures are intact. Sensation is WNL compared bil. DASH functional assessment score 28/100. Treatment today consisted of: 1) Education: HEP, activity modification, use of tennis elbow strap and 2) pulsed 1 MHz US @ 50% duty cycle 1.5 w/cm$^2$ x 8' to (L) lateral epicondyle, wrist extensor stretching with neutral and UD wrist, cross friction massage to extensor origin. Total exam time 30' and total tx time 20'.

**Plan of Care**: 35 y.o. male with medical dx of (L) lateral epicondylitis and PT dx: impaired mobility, function, muscle performance, and ROM due to local inflammation (Practice Pattern 4E). Pt. has good potential for improvement but recovery may require extended time due to chronic nature of injury. Skilled services are needed to administer modalities, friction massage, joint mobilizations, and teach pt. HEP, safe exercise progression, and activity modification. PT Impairments include: elbow pain and tenderness, decreased AROM (L) elbow, muscle weakness. Functional deficits include: decreased grip strength; painful work-related, home-management, and recreational tasks; limited in carrying heavy objects; and opening/closing jars (per DASH). PT intervention will consist of modalities, soft tissue massage, stretching, strengthening, and pt. education, including a HEP 2-3x/wk x 6-8 wks. Expected LTGs to be met by 8 wks: A.) Decrease pain 90-100%; B.) A/PROM (L) elbow WNL and pain free; C.) 5/5 strength (L) without pain; D.) Pain free grip strength = (R); E.) Pain-free work-related, home-management, and recreational tasks; F.) No difficulty in carrying heavy objects or opening/closing jars; G.) (I) with HEP. STGs to be met in 2 wks: A-1.) Decrease pain 10-20%; B-1.) Increase A/PROM by 5° for flexion and extension; C-1.) Strength 4+/5; D-1.) Increase pain free grip strength 10-15#; E-1.) Decrease pain during work-related, home-management, and recreational tasks by 50%; F-1.) Mild difficulty (per DASH) in carrying heavy objects or opening/closing jars; G-1.) (I) with initial stretching and activity modification. This pt. is in agreement with the plan of care.
Sue Smith, DPT

## Example 1B. Interim Note—Narrative Format

*PT Encounter*

**Patient**: John Smith
**Date of Service**: January 5, 2006 (Visit #2)

Pt. reports pain at level 6/10 at worst and 0 to 1/10 at best. Pain still increases with heavy grip, computer use, using hand tools. Reports compliance with HEP. No adverse effects from last tx. Palpable point tenderness on (L) lateral epicondyle and wrist extensor origin. AROM of (L) elbow is –10/140°. Treatment today consisted of: 1) pulsed 1 MHz US @ 50% duty cycle 1.5 w/cm$^2$ x 8′ to (L) lateral epicondyle; 2) wrist extensor stretching with neutral and UD wrist, cross friction massage to extensor origin and radiohumeral jt. mobilizations, grade 2; 3) Reviewed pt.'s HEP; and 4) Ice massage x 5′ to (L) extensor origin. (Total tx time 20′). Pt. notes slight improvement in pain since last visit. No other changes in objective or subjective data. Continue with current plan of care.
Sue Smith, DPT

## Example 1C. Reassessment—Narrative Format

**Patient**: John Smith
**Date of Service**: February 15, 2006 (Visit #12)

Pt. has been receiving PT since 1/3/06 for (L) lateral epicondylitis. Chief complaint at this time is still pain (3/10 at worst and 0/10 at best). It continues to increase with heavy grip and using hand tools. No longer having pain during work-related activities. Reporting primary functional deficits at this time include painful home management tasks and recreational activities. Global functional rating is 90% out of 100. Present therapy goals include returning to prior level of activity without pain and regaining all ROM. Musculoskeletal system shows palpable point tenderness on the (L) lateral epicondyle and wrist extensor origin. AROM of (L) elbow is –5/145° minimal to no pain at end range elbow flexion, extension, or wrist extension. MMT indicates (L) wrist extension and supination are 4+/5 with pain upon extension only. Continues to have (+) tennis elbow test. Pain free grip strength (R) 100, 110, 108#; (L) 85, 90, and 87#. DASH functional assessment score 13/100. Treatment today consisted of: 1) wrist extensor stretching with neutral and UD wrist, cross friction massage to extensor origin, eccentric strengthening to wrist extensors and supinators. Total re-exam time 30′ and tx time 30′.

**New Plan of Care**: PT dx: impaired mobility, function, muscle performance and ROM due to local inflammation (Practice Pattern 4E). Pt. continues to show good potential for improvement but has requires extended time due to chronic nature. Skilled services are needed to administer friction massage, joint mobilizations, safe exercise progression, and instruction in HEP. PT Impairments include: elbow pain and tenderness, decreased AROM (L) elbow, muscle weakness. Functional deficits include: decreased grip strength; painful home-management, and recreational tasks; limited in carrying heavy objects; and opening/closing jars. PT intervention will consist of modalities, soft tissue massage, stretching, strengthening, and pt. education, including a HEP 2-3x/wk x 6-8 wks. Expected LTGs to be met by 8 wks: A.) Decrease pain 90-100%; B.) A/PROM (L) elbow WNL and pain free; C.) 5/5 strength (L) without pain; D.) Pain free grip strength = (R); E.) Pain-free work-related, home-management, and recreational tasks; F.) No difficulty in carrying heavy objects or opening/closing jars; G.) (I) with HEP. STGs to be met in 2 wks: A-1.) Decrease pain 10-20% (Goal met); B-1.) Increase A/PROM by 5° for flexion and extension (Goal met); C-1.) Strength 4+/5 (Goal met); D-1.) Increase pain free grip strength 10-15# (Goal met); E-1.) Decrease pain during work-related, home-management, and recreational tasks by 50% (Goal met); F-1.) Mild difficulty (per DASH) in carrying heavy objects or opening/closing jars (Goal met); G-1.) (I) with initial stretching and activity modification (Goal met). For the next two weeks, we will continue to work toward meeting the above stated LTGs seeing the pt. 1-2x/wk (x2 wks). Tx will include: continued stretching, eccentric strengthening, jt. mobilizations, modalities if needed, and progression to return to normal activities. This pt. is in agreement with the new plan of care.
Sue Smith, DPT

## Example 1D. Discharge Summary—Narrative Format

*Discharge Summary*

**Patient**: John Smith
**Date**: March 10, 2006
**Dates of PT Services**: January 3 through March 10, 2006 (16 visits)

Present pain is 0/10 and occasionally goes to 1-2/10 with heavy gripping activities and prolonged use of hand tools. No pain with normal ADLs, home management, recreation, community or work activities. Denies activity limitations or participation restrictions. Global functional rating is 98/100. He reports that he can perform his HEP without difficulty and the "stretching has helped." Negative palpable point tenderness; AROM (L) elbow 0/145°; wrist extension and supination strength are 5/5 and pain free; (-) tennis elbow test; Pain free grip strength (R) 100, 110, 110# and (L) 98, 105, 100#; DASH functional score 8/100 (8%). Pt. has made good progress including improving AROM, MMT, and grip strength to normal. Also has shown reduced pain (90-100%) and improved function during normal ADLs, home management, work, community, and recreational activities (Initial DASH score 28/100, current 8/100). All LTGs have been met. Plan to d/c PT at this time to (I) HEP. Pt. will RTC if further problems arise. The pt. is in agreement with this plan.

## Example 1E—Other Narrative Examples

*Acute Care Setting*:

#1
02/9/06: Went to see pt. for gait & transfer training. Pt. lying in bed and reported feeling sick. Refused PT today. Jon Smith, PT

#2
05/3/06: Attempted to see pt. this p.m. Spoke with nursing prior to session, they indicated that pt. was to receive a blood transfusion and asked to withhold PT today. Will attempt to see pt. in a.m. if cleared. Jon Smith, PT

*Outpatient Setting*:
#1
04/5/06: Pt. called this morning reporting that she was not improving with therapy. Stated that she planned to call her physician. Canceled appointment for today. Will call to reschedule if needed. Jon Smith, PT

#2
Saw pt. today for follow-up visit after fabrication and fitting of (L) WHFO wrist cock-up splint. Remolded edge around thenar eminence and at MCP crease to allow more thumb and finger motion and decrease skin pressure at distal palmar crease. Pt. indicated improved motion with decreased pain after adjustment. Will have pt. return if needed for further splinting adjustments.
Jon Smith, PT

Table 4-1
## Common Headings Used to Add Structure to a Narrative Note

| Category Heading | Abbreviation |
|---|---|
| History of present illness | HPI |
| Mechanism of injury | MOI |
| Prior/Past Medical History | PMH |
| Chief complaint | c/c or C/C |
| Pain intensity or Pain rating | None |
| Lifestyle or Living situation | L/S or l/s |
| Strength | n/a |
| Range of motion | ROM |
| Functional Assessment | n/a |
| Interventions | n/a |
| Mobility | n/a |
| Gait | n/a (may see it abbreviated: gt.) |
| Transfers | n/a |
| PT diagnosis | PT dx |
| Short-term goals | STG |
| Long-term goals | LTG |
| Treatment Plan or Plan of care | Tx Plan |

## Example 2A. Initial Examination and Evaluation—POMR Format

*PT Examination and Evaluation*

**Patient**: John Smith
**Date of Service**: January 3, 2006

**Problem list**:
1. Elbow pain and point tenderness
2. Decreased AROM (L) elbow
3. Muscle weakness in (L) elbow, forearm, and wrist
4. Decreased grip strength
5. Painful work-related, home-management, and recreational tasks
6. Limited in carrying heavy objects and opening/closing jars

**Subjective**: Medical dx: (L) lateral epicondylitis; referred to PT by Dr. Jones

HPI: 35 y.o. male reports developing pain after spending the weekend painting his house 3 months ago. The pt. reports using ice and taking meds (OTC ibuprofen) initially but this didn't help. Saw his physician for a yearly physical and mentioned the elbow pain. His MD suggested "trying a few weeks of PT." Has not had any x-rays or imaging procedures. Pt. denies hx of a similar problem and prior elbow pain.

C/C: Pain (6/10 at worst and 2/10 at best) that increases with heavy grip, computer use, using hand tools. Denies temperature changes and numbness. Reports primary functional deficits include painful work-related activities, home management tasks, and recreational activities such as mountain biking and kayaking. Global functional rating is 85% out of 100.

PMH: Reports overall health is good with no relevant medical or surgical history.

L/S: Pt. lives alone and works as an accountant.

Pt.'s Goals: Pain reduction allowing improvement in functional tasks and prevention of recurrence.

**Objective**: Gross ROS: BP: 120/84, HR: 78 bpm, and RR: 12. Neurological and integumentary systems are not impaired. No impairments in cognitive or communicative status. Impairments noted in musculoskeletal system.

Pain: Musculoskeletal system shows palpable point tenderness on the (L) lateral epicondyle and wrist extensor origin.

AROM: (R) UE is WNL (elbow 0/145°); (L) shoulder, wrist, and hand are WNL except elbow is –10/140; c/o pain at end range elbow flexion, extension, and wrist extension; cervical A/PROM also WNL and pain free.

PROM: (L) elbow is 0/145 with normal end feel but c/o pain.

*(continued)*

## Example 2A. Initial Examination and Evaluation—POMR Format, continued

Strength: MMT indicates 5/5 strength throughout (B) UE except (L) wrist extension and supination are 4/5 with pain. All provocation tests for (L) elbow are unremarkable except a (+) tennis elbow test. Pain free grip strength (R) 100, 110, 108#; (L) 65, 60, 55# with pain.

Anthropometric measurements: (-) edema compared bil.

Neurovascular: Neurovascular structures are intact. Sensation is WNL compared bil.

Function: DASH functional assessment score 28/100. Most difficulty with carrying heavy objects and opening/closing jars (see attached).

Time: Exam: 30'

Imp: PT dx: impaired mobility, function, muscle performance and ROM due to local inflammation (Practice Pattern 4E). Pt. has good potential for improvement but may require extended time for recovery due to chronic nature. Skilled services are needed to administer modalities, friction massage, joint mobilizations, and teach pt. HEP, safe exercise progression, and activity modification.

Expected LTGs: to be met by 8 wks: A.) Decrease pain 90-100%; B.) A/PROM (L) elbow WNL and pain free; C.) 5/5 strength (L) without pain; D.) Pain free grip strength = (R); E.) Pain-free work-related, home-management, and recreational tasks; F.) No difficulty in carrying heavy objects or opening/closing jars; G.) (I) with HEP.

STGs to be met in 2 wks: A-1.) Decrease pain 10-20%; B-1.) Increase A/PROM by 5° for flexion and extension; C-1.) Strength 4+/5; D-1.) Increase pain free grip strength 10-15#; E-1.) Decrease pain during work-related, home-management, and recreational tasks by 50%; F-1.) Mild difficulty (per DASH) in carrying heavy objects or opening/closing jars; G-1.) (I) with initial stretching and activity modification.

**Tx today**: 1) Education: HEP, activity modification, use of tennis elbow strap and 2) pulsed 1 MHz US @ 50% duty cycle 1.5 w/cm$^2$ x 8' to (L) lateral epicondyle, wrist extensor stretching with neutral and UD wrist, cross friction massage to extensor origin. Tx time: 20'

**Plan**: PT interventions will consist of modalities, soft tissue massage, stretching, strengthening, and pt. education, including a HEP 2-3x/wk x 6-8 wks.

This pt. is in agreement with the plan of care.

Sue Smith, DPT

## Example 2B. Interim Note—POMR Format

*A separate entry for each problem is completed; therefore for this date of service, there would be potentially six entries in to the chart. Two entries are provided as examples using this format.*

**Patient**: John Smith
**Date of Service**: January 3, 2006
**Current problems**:
1. Elbow pain and point tenderness
2. Decreased AROM (L) elbow
3. Muscle weakness
4. Decreased grip strength
5. Painful work-related, home-management, and recreational tasks
6. Limited in carrying heavy objects and opening/closing jars (per DASH)

**Note for Problem #1—Elbow pain and point tenderness:**
S: Pt. reports pain at level 6/10 at worst and 0 to 1/10 at best. Pain still increases with heavy grip, computer use, using hand tools. Reports compliance with HEP.
O: Palpable point tenderness on (L) lateral epicondyle and wrist extensor origin.
Imp.: Pt. notes slight improvement in pain since last visit. No other changes in objective or subjective data.
Tx: Treatment today consisted of: 1) pulsed 1 MHz US @ 50% duty cycle 1.5 w/cm$^2$ x 8' to (L) lateral epicondyle; 2) Reviewed pt.'s HEP; and 4) Ice massage x 5' to (L) extensor origin. (Total tx time 20').
Plan: Continue with current plan of care.
Sue Smith, DPT

---

**Example 2B. Interim Note—POMR Format, continued**

**Note for Problem #2—Decreased AROM (L) elbow:**
S: No subjective comments on ROM
O: AROM of (L) elbow is –10/140°.
Imp.: No changes in ROM since initial visit.
Tx: Treatment today consisted of: 1) wrist extensor stretching with neutral and UD wrist, cross friction massage to extensor origin and radiohumeral jt. mobilizations, grade 2
Plan: Continue with current plan of care.
Sue Smith, DPT

---

- Allows a clinician who is interested in a particular problem to go directly to that aspect of the note, thus easing communication among care providers

- Provides a chronological sequence of interventions for a particular problem, better outlining the problem-solving process

Regardless of the benefits to the structure provided with the POMR, authors have reported problems with it as well. First, the POMR separates, or fragments patients according to their problems. Because of this, providers may not see the "whole patient."[3] For example, in more complex cases, it is possible that a clinician working with breathing might not be aware of postural problems without reading separate chart entries. Yet reading all chart entries for each problem could be very time consuming. In addition, for patients with multiple problems, the POMR can become increasingly complex requiring an extraordinary amount of time for an individual managing multiple problems.

In the mid 1970s, several authors reported on the use of the POMR in rehabilitation.[4-6,8,9] Reinstein et al[9] supplemented the POMR with the Rehabilitation Evaluation System that included scoring the patient's ability to perform 18 functional activities. Later, they reported that this form of documentation in the rehabilitation setting improved communication among team members, but it was too complex for complicated patients that are often encountered.[6]

## SOAP Notes

*SOAP* is an acronym for subjective, objective, assessment, and plan. The SOAP format evolved from the POMR initially described by Weed. Like in the POMR, "S", or subjective, should include anything the patient tells you pertaining to his or her injuries or illness. Subjective information can also be any information provided by the patient's family or caregivers. The "O," or objective section includes relevant tests and measurements performed, the patient's functional status, and physical therapy interventions performed for that day of service. Unlike the POMR, in the SOAP

format, the physical therapy interventions are written in the objective portion of the note, and the interpretation, or impression, has been designated "A, " for assessment. In the SOAP format, the "P" stands for plan. Specific information provided in the S, O, A, and P portions of the notes can be found in Figures 4-1 through 4-4.

Unlike the POMR, one "SOAP note," as it is often called, includes information pertaining to all of the patient's problems. The SOAP note may or may not be preceded by a "Problem" (Pr:) section. When used, the "Problem" section contains information pertaining to the medical diagnosis and/or referral information (Example 3A). You will read more about the "Problem" and SOAP in subsequent chapters.

The SOAP format is now widely used by a variety of medical and rehabilitation professionals. The SOAP note has become a stand-alone format for documentation and is used for initial documentation (Example 3A), interim and/or progress notes (Example 3B), re-evaluations or reassessments (Example 3C), and discharge summaries (Example 3D). Like the POMR, SOAP note documentation provides structure to medical record entries. In addition, SOAP notes show logical decision-making by using subjective and objective information to determine an assessment and plan.

While SOAP notes provide a consistent, concise format for documenting the patient's subjective remarks, objective exam findings, the provider's overall impression, and the plan of care, more recently, it has been scrutinized. Several reasons for this scrutiny exist. First, subjective documentation is often centered around the patient's complaints, primarily pain. Second, objective findings are often written in terms of impairments, such as range of motion, strength, balance, etc. Assessments are often written in terms of how the patient tolerated the treatment, ie, "Tolerated treatment well." Furthermore, the relationship between improvements in the patient's impairments and improved functional capabilities are usually implied or assumed, rather than described in specific detail with reference to objective data.[10,11] Additionally, the relationship between interventions and improvement are also implied rather than explained. These problems often result in documentation centered on the patient's complaints and

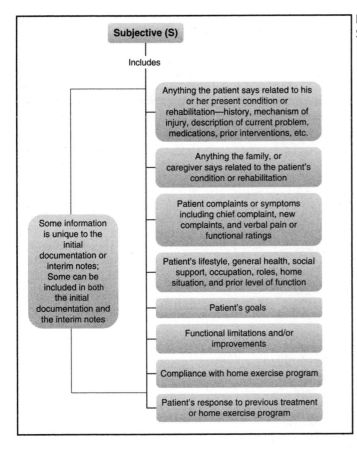

**Figure 4-1.** Subjective data found in the "S" portion of a SOAP note.

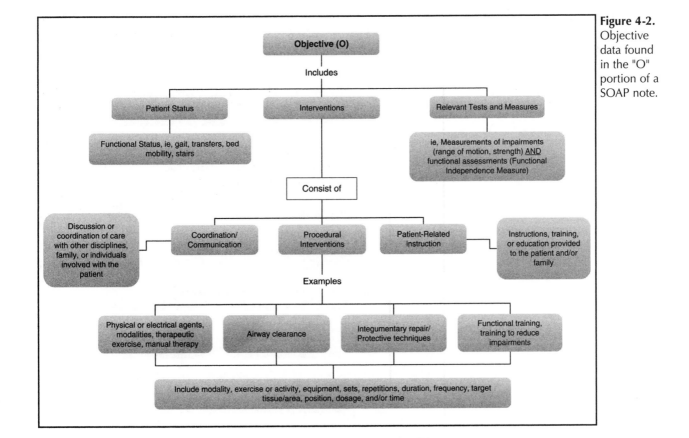

**Figure 4-2.** Objective data found in the "O" portion of a SOAP note.

**Figure 4-3.** Information found in the "A" portion of a SOAP note.

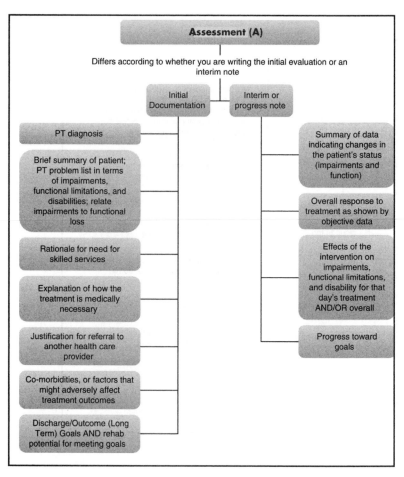

**Figure 4-4.** Information found in the "P" portion of a SOAP note.

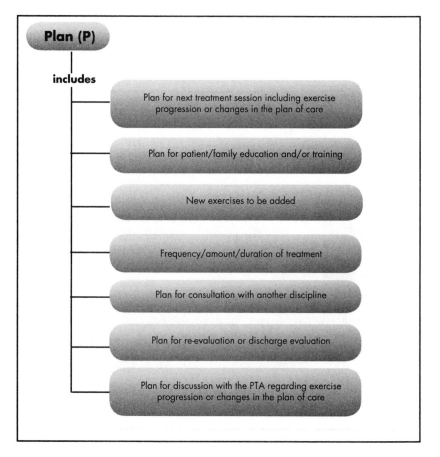

## Example 3A. Initial Examination and Evaluation—SOAP Format

*PT Examination and Evaluation*

**Patient**: John Smith
**Date of Service**: January 3, 2006

**Pr**: <u>Medical dx</u>: (L) lateral epicondylitis; referred to PT by Dr. Jones
**S**: <u>HPI</u>: 35 y.o. male reports developing pain after spending the weekend painting his house 3 months ago. The pt. reports using ice and taking meds (OTC ibuprofen) initially but this didn't help. Saw his physician for a yearly physical and mentioned the elbow pain. His MD suggested "trying a few weeks of PT." Has not had any x-rays or imaging procedures. Pt. denies hx of a similar problem and prior elbow pain.
<u>C/C</u>: Pain (6/10 at worst and 2/10 at best) that increases with heavy grip, computer use, using hand tools. Denies temperature changes and numbness. Reports primary functional deficits include painful work-related activities, home management tasks, and recreational activities such as mountain biking and kayaking. Global functional rating is 85% out of 100.
<u>PMH</u>: Reports overall health is good with no relevant medical or surgical history.
<u>L/S</u>: Pt. lives alone and works as an accountant.
<u>Pt.'s Goals</u>: Pain reduction allowing improvement in functional tasks and prevention of recurrence.
**O**: <u>Gross ROS</u>: BP: 120/84, HR: 78 bpm, and RR: 12. Neurological and integumentary systems are not impaired. No impairments in cognitive or communicative status. Impairments noted in musculoskeletal system, see below.
<u>Pain</u>: Musculoskeletal system shows palpable point tenderness on the (L) lateral epicondyle and wrist extensor origin.
<u>AROM</u>: (R) UE is WNL (elbow 0/145°); (L) shoulder, wrist, and hand are WNL except elbow is –10/140; c/o pain at end range elbow flexion, extension, and wrist extension; cervical A/PROM also WNL and pain free.
<u>PROM</u>: (L) elbow is 0/145 with normal end feel but c/o pain.
<u>Strength</u>: MMT indicates 5/5 strength throughout (B) UE except (L) wrist extension and supination are 4/5 with pain. All special provocation tests for (L) elbow are unremarkable except a (+) tennis elbow test. Pain free grip strength (R) 100, 110, 108#; (L) 65, 60, 55# with pain.
<u>Anthropometric measurements</u>: (-) edema compared bil.
<u>Neurovascular</u>: Neurovascular structures are intact. Sensation is WNL compared bil.
<u>Function</u>: DASH functional assessment score 28/100. Most difficulty with carrying heavy objects and opening and closing jars (see attached).
<u>Tx today</u>: 1) Education: HEP, activity modification, use of tennis elbow strap and 2) pulsed 1 MHz US @ 50% duty cycle 1.5 w/cm$^2$ x 8' to (L) lateral epicondyle, wrist extensor stretching with neutral and UD wrist, cross friction massage to extensor origin. <u>Time</u>: Exam: 30'; Tx: 20'; Total: 50'.
**A**: PT dx: impaired mobility, function, muscle performance and ROM due to local inflammation (Practice Pattern 4E).
<u>Rehab Potential</u>: Good potential for improvement but may require extended time due to chronic nature of the injury and teach pt. HEP, safe exercise progression, and activity modification.
<u>PT Impairments</u>: elbow pain and tenderness, decreased AROM (L) elbow, muscle weakness.
<u>Functional deficits</u>: include: decreased grip strength; painful work-related, home-management, and recreational tasks; limited in carrying heavy objects; and opening/closing jars.
<u>Expected LTGs</u>: to be met by 8 wks:
A) Decrease pain 90-100%;
B) A/PROM (L) elbow WNL and pain free;
C) 5/5 strength (L) without pain;
D) Pain free grip strength = (R);
E) Pain-free work-related, home-management, and recreational tasks;
F) No difficulty in carrying heavy objects or opening/closing jars
G) (I) with HEP.
<u>STGs</u>: to be met in 2 wks:
A-1) Decrease pain 10-20%;
B-1) Increase A/PROM by 5° for flexion and extension;
C-1) Strength 4+/5;
D-1) Increase pain free grip strength 10-15#;
E-1) Decrease pain during work-related, home-management, and recreational tasks by 50%;
F-1) Mild difficulty (per DASH) in carrying heavy objects or opening/closing jars;
G-1) (I) with initial stretching and activity modification.

*(continued)*

## Example 3A. Initial Examination and Evaluation—SOAP Format, continued

**P**: PT interventions will consist of modalities, soft tissue massage, stretching, strengthening, and pt. education, including a HEP 2-3x/wk x 6-8 wks.
This pt. is in agreement with the plan of care.
Sue Smith, DPT

## Example 3B. Interim Note—SOAP Format

**Patient**: John Smith
**Date of Service**: January 5, 2006 (Visit #2)

**S**: Pt. reports pain at level 6/10 at worst and 0 to 1/10 at best. Pain still increases with heavy grip, computer use, using hand tools. Reports compliance with HEP. No adverse effects from last tx.
**O**: Palpable point tenderness on (L) lateral epicondyle and wrist extensor origin. <u>AROM</u>: (L) elbow is –10/140 .
<u>Treatment today</u>: 1) pulsed 1 MHz US @ 50% duty cycle 1.5 w/cm² x 8' to (L) lateral epicondyle; 2) wrist extensor stretching with neutral and UD wrist, cross friction massage to extensor origin and radiohumeral jt. mobilizations, grade 2; 3) Reviewed pt.'s HEP; and 4) Ice massage x 5' to (L) extensor origin. (Total tx time 20').
**A**: Pt. notes slight improvement in pain since last visit (0-1/10 versus 2/10). No other changes in objective or subjective data.
**P**: Continue with current plan of care.
Sue Smith, DPT

## Example 3C. Reassessment—SOAP Format

**Patient**: John Smith
**Date of Service**: February 15, 2006 (Visit #12)

**Pr.**: PT since 1/3/06 for (L) lateral epicondylitis.
**S**: <u>C/C</u>: pain (3/10 at worst and 0/10 at best). It continues to increase with increases with heavy grip and using hand tools. No longer having pain during work-related activities. <u>Functional status</u>: Reporting primary functional deficits at this time include painful home management tasks and recreational activities. Global functional rating is 90% out of 100.
<u>Pt.'s goals</u>: Present therapy goals include returning to prior level of activity without pain and regaining all ROM.
**O**: Musculoskeletal system shows palpable point tenderness on the (L) lateral epicondyle and wrist extensor origin.
<u>AROM</u>: (L) elbow –5/145° with minimal to no pain at end range elbow flexion, extension, or wrist extension.
<u>Strength</u> : (L) wrist extension and supination are 4+/5 & pain with extension only, ie, (+) tennis elbow test. Pain free grip strength (R) 100, 110, 108# (L) 85, 90, and 87#.
<u>Functional assessment</u>: DASH functional assessment score 13/100.
<u>Today's tx</u>: 1) wrist extensor stretching with neutral and UD wrist, cross friction massage to extensor origin, eccentric strengthening to wrist extensors and supinators. Total re-exam time 30' and tx time 30'.
**A**: <u>PT dx</u>: impaired mobility, function, muscle performance and ROM due to local inflammation (Practice Pattern 4E). Pt. continues to show good potential for improvement. Skilled services are needed to administer friction massage, joint mobilizations, and teach pt. safe exercise progression, and HEP.
<u>PT Impairments</u>: elbow pain and tenderness, decreased AROM (L) elbow, muscle weakness.
<u>Functional limitations</u>: decreased grip strength; painful home-management and recreational tasks; limited in carrying heavy objects; and opening/closing jars.

*(continued)*

## Example 3C. Re-Examination and Re-Evaluation—SOAP Format, continued

Expected LTGs to be met in next 2 wks:
- A) Decrease pain 90-100%;
- B) A/PROM (L) elbow WNL and pain free;
- C) 5/5 strength (L) without pain;
- D) Pain free grip strength = (R);
- E) Pain-free work-related, home-management, and recreational tasks;
- F) No difficulty in carrying heavy objects or opening/closing jars;
- G) (I) with HEP.

STGs from initial evaluation:
- A-1) Decrease pain 10-20% (Goal met);
- B-1) Increase A/PROM by 5° for flexion and extension (Goal met);
- C-1) Strength 4+/5 (Goal met);
- D-1) Increase pain free grip strength 10-15# (Goal met);
- E-1) Decrease pain during work-related, home-management, and recreational tasks by 50% (Goal met);
- F-1) Mild difficulty (per DASH) in carrying heavy objects or opening/closing jars (Goal met);
- G-1) (I) with initial stretching and activity modification (Goal met).

**P**: PT intervention will consist of modalities, soft tissue massage, stretching, strengthening, and pt. education, including a HEP. For the next two weeks, we will continue to work toward meeting the above stated LTGs seeing the pt. 1-2x. Tx will include: continued stretching, eccentric strengthening, joint mobilizations, modalities if needed, and progression to return to normal activities. This pt. is in agreement with the new plan of care.
Sue Smith, DPT

---

## Example 3D. Discharge Summary—SOAP Format

**Pt**: John Smith
**Date**: March 10, 2006

**Dates of PT Services**: January 3 through March 10, 2006 (16 visits)
**Pr**: (L) lateral epicondylitis
**S**: C/C: At present pain is 0/10 and occasionally goes to 1-2/10 with heavy activities like using hand tools. No pain with normal ADLs, home management, recreation, community or work activities. Denies activity limitations or participation restrictions. Global functional rating is 98/100. He reports that he can perform his HEP without difficulty and the "stretching has helped."
**O**: Pain: Negative palpable point tenderness; AROM: (L) elbow 0/145°; Strength: wrist extension and supination strength are 5/5 and pain free; (-) tennis elbow test; Pain free grip strength (R) 100, 110, 110# and (L) 98, 105, 100#; Function: DASH functional score 8/100 (8%).
**A**: Pt. has made good progress including improving AROM, MMT, and grip strength to WNL. Also has shown reduced pain (90-100%) and improved function during normal ADLs, home management, work, community, and recreational activities (Initial DASH score 28/100, current 8/100). LTGs: All have been met.
**P**: d/c PT at this time to (I) HEP. Pt. will RTC if further problems arise. Pt. is in agreement with this plan.
Sue Smith, PT

impairments, rather than progress toward functional restoration. An emerging problem with the SOAP format is that the writer often leaves out explaining the need for skilled services and a description of why treatment is medically necessary. Nevertheless, the SOAP format is widely acceptable and can be an appropriate form of documentation if its emphasis shifts toward linking impairments, function, and interventions.

## Functional Outcome Reporting (FOR)

Functional outcome reporting (FOR) emerged in the early 1990s and is becoming more popular in rehabilitation. Quinn and Gordon[1] described FOR as a type of documentation that focuses on the ability to perform meaningful functional activities rather than isolated musculoskeletal, neuromuscular, cardiopulmonary, or integumentary impairments. Advantages of FOR have been identified. The FOR format establishes a relationship between the patient's impairments and the ability to perform functional tasks, and it improves readability for non-health care providers reviewing documentation.[1,12]

While the importance of integrating impairments with function has been provided in preceding sections, the SOAP format is still the most common type of documentation used in physical therapy practice with functional skills being reported as part of the SOAP note. Authors have suggested combining FOR with the SOAP format.[12,13] When combining FOR with the SOAP format, Abeln[12] suggested the making the following additions to SOAP:

1. Objective (O) section:

   - Clearly and objectively provide the patient's prior and current functional status, including functional activities that are specific to that patient

2. Assessment (A) section:
   - List only those impairments being addressed with therapy
   - Describe how improvement in impairments will lead to improvement in functional limitations
   - Provide complicating factors, eg, co-morbidities

- PTs write goals using functional terminology

Examples 3A through 3D are written in a manner to show integration of FOR and SOAP.

This chapter outlines several different reasons and ways to document patient/client management. In clinical practice, you are likely to encounter a wide variety of documentation styles, and it is important that you adhere to your facility's approved format as well as state and federal laws. It is the authors' experience that the POMR is least prevalent while the SOAP format is most widely used; however, language describing the patient's prior and current functional status is becoming more common. Narrative notes also serve distinct purposes as previously described. Although there is no evidence suggesting superiority of one type of note over another, you will soon find that in real-world clinical practice, you are likely to apply principles from the three latter types, thus using a combination of narrative, SOAP, and FOR. Regardless of the structure, documentation of the patient's prior, current, and required functional levels is imperative.

The authors of this text have selected the basic SOAP structure to provide a framework for learning documentation skills. You will be exposed to information that should go into the "S," "O," "A," and "P" portions of the note. In addition, you will be exposed to how aspects of the patient/client management model can fit into the SOAP format (Table 4-2). The SOAP structure was selected because of its prevalence in clinical practice, and because of its adaptability to a variety of documentation styles and settings. Regardless of the format, well-written records include pertinent subjective and objective data (including functional status) that justify a reasonable and medically necessary plan of care. Well-written records are necessary for reimbursement, and therefore quality must be a priority.

In addition to structuring a note, this text will expose you to including a disablement model into your documentation, thus further emphasizing what the patient can and cannot do from a functional standpoint. The following points will be emphasized throughout: 1) linking impairments to functional deficits; 2) linking interventions to their effects on impairments and function; and 3) showing how a reduction of impairments allows improved function and participation in normal life roles and tasks.

| Table 4-2 | | | |
|---|---|---|---|
| *Correlation Between Information in the Patient/Client Management Model and SOAP Format* | | | |
| Component of Patient/Client Management | Includes: | What to record: | Where information is found when using the "SOAP" format |
| Examination | 1) History | • Subjective data | "S" OR SUBJECTIVE SECTION |
| | 2) Systems review: Cardiovascular System Integumentary System Musculoskeletal System Neuromuscular System Cognitive/Communicative ability 3) Tests and measures | • Objective data—Results of systems review and tests and measures | "O" OR OBJECTIVE SECTION |
| Evaluation | Clinical judgment, problem-solving process, determining PT diagnosis and prognosis, and establishing the plan of care | • Brief summary of the patient, synthesizing exam findings, including relation-ship between impairments and function<br>• Need for referral to another health care provider<br>• PT problems and need for skilled services<br>• Factors influencing treat-ment (ie, co-morbidities)<br>• PT diagnosis (Can use ICD-9 or a practice pattern from the *Guide to PT Practice*)<br>• Rehab potential<br>• Physical therapy goals | "A" OR ASSESSMENT |
| | | • Planned interventions including frequency, duration, and amount of treatment<br>• Discharge plans | "P" OR PLAN |
| (Reference: American Physical Therapy Association. Defensible documentation. Available at: http://www.apta.org/AM/Template.cfm?Section=Home&NAVMENUID=2505&CONTENTID=37071&DIRECTLISTCOMBOIND=D&TEMPLATE=/MembersOnly.cfm. Accessed July 30, 2007.) | | | |

## Review Questions

1. What are similarities and differences between narrative notes, SOAP notes, POMR, and FOR?

2. What are advantages and disadvantages of narrative notes, SOAP notes, POMR, and FOR?

3. Give examples of information you would find in the S, O, A, and P portions of the note.

4. What is the importance of documenting a patient's functional status?

5. What ways can a patient's functional status be written into a SOAP note?

6. How can elements of the Patient/Client Management Model be integrated into a SOAP note?

7. List information written as part of the evaluation, PT diagnosis, and PT prognosis. How are they included/written into a SOAP note?

8. Name important information that should be included in a Plan of Care. How are plan of care requirements integrated into SOAP format?

9. Which format (Narrative, POMR, SOAP, FOR) is best for documenting unexpected or unusual circumstances?

## Application Exercises

I. Read the following statements and determine if it would belong in the S, O, A, or P portions of a SOAP note.

_____ Gait: Ambulated 50' x 2 WBAT ℝ LE c̄ min@ x 1 & verbal cues to advance ℝ LE

_____ Pt. reports HEP has helped ↑ ROM

_____ Pt. will RTC 2x/wk x 4 wks

_____ Transfers: bed ↔ chair c̄ mod @ x 2

_____ Pt. progressing toward goals set on the initial evaluation

_____ Pt.'s wife stated that she has been assisting the pt. c̄ his HEP

_____ Speak c̄ the MD about ↓ in BP upon transferring supine → sit

_____ AROM: ℝ knee 0-135°

_____ Improvements in knee AROM allow pt. to sit s̄ difficulty and ↓ ↑ stairs c̄ less difficulty

_____ Pt. reports that he is benefiting from the strengthening exercises in that he is now able to open jars and lids (I)

_____ Pt. will be seen for bid gait training

_____ Pt. c/o inability to move her (L) UE and LE

_____ Pt. denies use of assistive device prior to admission

_____ Gait distance improved from 25' to 150' over the last week

_____ Pt. demonstrating (L) neglect making her unsafe during gait & transfers

_____ Muscle Performance: All (R) LE strength is 5/5

_____ Vitals: HR 95 bpm, RR 12, BP 140/95

_____ Pt. has improved ability to transfer in/out of bed since initial visit

_____ Will contact MD about possible d/c as pt. is no longer benefiting from the interventions

_____ Pt.'s endurance is poor 2° to COPD

_____ Pt. c/o inability to brush teeth and eat c̄ (R) hand 2° to ↓ AROM of the (R) elbow

_____ Pt. is unable to drive or perform safe community mobility at this time

_____ Edema in (R) ankle has ↓ 2 cm.

_____ Pt. dons/doffs prosthesis (I)

_____ Wound appearance: 100% red, healthy granulation tissue c̄ minimal drainage

- Of the above statements, which would be considered "functional" and would be considered appropriate using the FOR?

- Of the above, which would you consider to be integrating treatment, impairments, and function?

II. You are a physical therapy student in a neurological rehabilitation hospital. You are assigned to work with a patient with the following problems:

- Flaccid (complete paralysis) left upper extremity

- Weakness in left lower extremity

- Dependence with ambulation

- Requires assist for all transfers

- Unable to perform self-care or home management skills

1. List three questions that you could ask this patient when initiating a treatment session to elicit information for the subjective portion of a SOAP note.

2. What are three tests, measurements, or functional activities you could objectively perform and document for this patient?

3. Compare and contrast use of the SOAP note, POMR, and FOR for this patient. What would be the same in all three? What would be different? Which of these documentation formats would be most difficult to complete for this patient?

III. Read through the following initial examination/evaluation and answer the questions that follow.

**Date**: March 1, 2004
**Pr**: 27 y.o. male s/p (L) wrist & ankle fx; Referred to OP PT to begin gentle wrist & ankle AROM & PROM; May begin using cx c̄ platform for (L) UE. PWB 50% (L) LE
**S**: HPI: 4 wks. s/p fall (~25′) from a logging truck landing on his (L) side (2/1/04). Pt. sustained fx of the (L) distal radius and ulna & (L) distal tibia & fibula. Pt. underwent ORIF for the wrist and ankle immediately after the injury. He was placed in a SAC for the UE and SLC for the LE. He was NWB on the (L) LE & has been unable to use cx 2° to not being allowed to bear weight on the affected UE. At the time of the fall, the pt. also sustained a mild concussion. He was hospitalized for 5 days following the injury. While hospitalized he received IP PT to learn how to negotiate his w/c & transfer in/out bed. Both casts were removed yesterday & his ankle was placed in a removable splint. Reports taking ibuprofen PRN for pain
C/C: Pain & stiffness in (L) UE & LE c̄ ↓ functional use of (B). Doesn't like using w/c for mobility. Unable to work. Requiring assist c̄ self-care activities & home management
L/S: RHD; Lives c̄ wife & 2 small children in single level home c̄ 2 steps @ entrance & HR on the (R). Prior to injury pt. was employed as a construction worker. He has been off work since the DOI. Pt. is unable to drive & is relying on his wife & mother for transportation. No significant PMH or hx of fx. Reports being a non-smoker and non-drinker. Family hx is + for OA.
Pt's Goals: Return to previous level of function and RTW ASAP. Learn to ambulate c̄ cx.
**O**: AROM: (R) UE & LE WNL; (L) shoulder, elbow, & hip WNL

| L wrist: | AROM | PROM |
|---|---|---|
| Flexion | 20° | 25° |
| Extension | 10° | 15° |
| UD | 10° | 15° |
| RD | 15° | 15° |
| Supination | 30° | 35° |
| Pronation | 40° | 45° |

L hand: Pt. can perform a full fist but it is difficult 2° to edema; Thumb IP, MCP, and CMC AROM is WNL

| L knee: | 0-100° | 0-110° |
|---|---|---|
| L ankle: | | |
| DF | -10 from neutral | 0° (neutral) |
| PF | 20° | 25° |
| Inv | 5° | 5° |
| Ev | 0° | 5° |

Strength: (R) UE & LE 5/5; (L) shoulder and hip 4/5; (L) elbow, wrist, knee, & ankle deferred 2° to acuity
Girth: wrist figure 8 (R): 36 cm (L): 37.2 cm; ankle figure 8 (R): 42 cm (L): 44.1 cm Sensation: (L) wrist & ankle intact to light touch & (=) when compared to (R)
Circulation: 2+ at radial & dorsal pedal arteries on the (L) Special Tests: N/A @ this time 2° acuity
Gait: Unable to ambulate at this time
Transfers: (I) bed ↔ chair, chair ↔ toilet, sit ↔ stand all NWB on (L) LE
Bed Mobility: (I) all areas.
Tx & HEP: AROM & PROM for (L) wrist: flexion, extension, pronation, & supination; (L) ankle: DF& PF (also instructed in using opposite foot for self PROM); performed AROM for all digits and thumb; instructed pt. in using ice, elevation & compression wrapping for ankle and wrist; instructed pt. in use of cx c̄ platform for (L) UE, PWB 50% on (L) LE using step to gait pattern. Pt. required CGA x 1 for balance c̄ cx & gait pattern. Pt. performed all ex. (I) & verbalized understanding of all precautions. Total treatment time 45′ following exam.
**A**: 27 y.o. RHD female 4 wks s/p fall. Now c̄ impaired mobility due to fractures. Demonstrating ↓ AROM, PROM, & strength. Unable to ambulate, perform self-care or home management tasks s̄ assistance. Unable to work @ this time. Skilled services necessary to instruct pt. in appropriate ROM ex., use of AD & progress gait as ordered. Also will require instruction in strengthening exercises, and retraining in functional mobility to prepare for return to normal L/S and RTW. Pt. able to communicate s̄ limitations & demonstrates good potential for full recovery. No co-morbidities that could affect outcome identified at this time.

*Anticipated Goals and Expected Outcomes*:
At the end of 2 weeks, the pt. will:
1. Increase AROM 10-15° for the wrist, forearm, and ankle
2. Decrease edema by .5 cm for the wrist and ankle
3. Ambulate c̄ cx c̄ (L) UE platform PWB (L) LE (I)
4. Perform all self-care (I)
5. Perform a full fist s̄ limitations

At the end of 16 weeks (d/c), the pt. will:
1. Have normal AROM of the wrist, forearm, & ankle (90-100% of opposite)
2. Grip & pinch strength will be 80-100% of ®
3. Be (I) c̄ all self-care & home management tasks
4. Ambulate (I) on all surfaces s̄ use of AD
5. ↑↓ flight of stairs (I) s̄ AD
6. Drive s̄ restrictions
7. RTW @ previous level of employment

**P**: See pt. 3x/wk for next 3-4 mos. to work on AROM & PROM of the wrist and ankle, strengthening ex. for the hip, knee, shoulder and elbow, gait training, functional mobility, & progress strengthening of the involved extremities when appropriate. Will progress pt. as tolerated & according to MD orders. Pt. is in agreement c̄ the above stated plan.
John Smith, PT

1. What note writing format is being used?
2. List 3 pieces of subjective data found in the note.
3. List 3 pieces of objective data found in the note.
4. What information is found in the A and P portions of the note?
5. Write a problem list for this patient that includes all movement-related impairments.
6. Write a problem list for this patient that includes all functional limitations/disabilities (NAGI).
7. Write a problem list for this patient that includes all activity limitations (ICF) (performance without assistance).
8. Write a problem list for this patient that includes all movement-related participation restrictions (ICF) (actual performance).
9. In what part of the note (S, O, A, or P) would you place a problem list? Why?
10. Would you consider this patient to be disabled? Why or why not.
11. How did the PT describe the need for skilled care?

12. On the next visit with the patient, what information or data would you need to collect and record in an interim note for this patient to show changes in status or progress for the initial session?
13. In an interim note, in what section (S, O, A, or P) would you explain the changes in the patient's status?
14. What would be the most appropriate format for the interim note? Explain your answer.
15. Is this patient's care medically necessary? Why or why not? What evidence is there of medical necessity?
16. What other providers/individuals might be interested in looking at this patient's note(s)?

IV.  Read the following patient information:

*Number 1*:

You are working with an elderly female in the acute hospital setting who has suffered a (R) CVA. The patient is cooperative and has no complaints. You performed passive and active assisted range of motion to the patient's left extremities. The patient was not showing any signs of abnormal tone or signs of developing contractures. You performed 3 sets of

10 repetitions. You also provided manual resistance to the patient's right lower extremity. The patient tolerated two sets of 10 repetitions for the resisted range of motion. Finally you provided stretching to the patient's tight ankle plantarflexors. You provided the stretch 5 times for each side holding each stretch for 30 seconds each. You will continue the same treatment the following day and progress as tolerated.

A. Organize the information into a narrative note.

B. Organize the information into a SOAP note.

*Number 2:*

You are working with an in-patient with Guillain Barre Syndrome. He reports that he is doing better today. Exercises consisted of ankle pumps, active hip abduction, heel slides, bridging, and knee extension at the edge of the bed 3 sets of 10 reps. After exercises, you worked on transfers to the wheelchair that was positioned next to the bed using a stand pivot, the patient required about 25-30% assistance from you, but you were able to provide this yourself without difficulty. Although you did have to block his knees so they did not buckle due to weakness. After this, the patient transferred back to bed, but because of fatigue and bed height, he requires 50-60% assist. He performed sit to and from supine with 50% assistance because of weakness. He was unable to lift his legs onto the bed from the floor. He was able to position himself in bed without the use of side rails while scooting and bridging with verbal cues. There was no improvement in the patient's ability to transfer from the previous day's note. You tell him you will see him in the afternoon for gait in the department.

A. Organize the information into a narrative note.

B. Organize the information into a SOAP note.

# References

1. Quinn L, Gordon J. *Functional outcomes: Documentation for rehabilitation.* St. Louis, MO: Saunders; 2003.
2. Weed LL. *Medical Records, Medical Education, and Patient Care: The Problem-Oriented Medical Record as a Basic Tool.* Chicago, IL: Year Book Medical Publishers; 1970.
3. Feinstein AR. The problems of the 'problem-oriented medical record'. *Ann Intern Med.* 1973;78(5):751-62.
4. Dinsdale SM, Mossman PL, Gullickson G, Anderson TP. The problem-oriented medical record in rehabilitation. *Arch Phys Med Rehabil.* 1970;51(8):488-92.
5. Milhous RL. The problem-oriented medical record in rehabilitation management and training. *Arch Phys Med Rehabil.* 1972;53(4):182-5.
6. Reinstein L. Problem-oriented medical record: experience in 238 rehabilitation institutions. *Arch Phys Med Rehabil.* 1977;58(9):398-401.
7. Mcintyre N. The problem-oriented medical record. *Br Med J.* 1973;2(5866):598-600.
8. Grabois M. The problem-oriented medical record: modification and simplification for rehabilitation medicine. *South Med J.* 1977;70(11):1383-5.
9. Reinstein L, Staas WE, Marquette CH. A rehabilitation evaluation system which complements the problem-oriented medical record. *Arch Phys Med Rehabil.* 1975;56(9):396-9.
10. White JA. Managing care. Documentation: making it meaningful. *Physical Therapy Case Reports.* 2000;3(2):78-9.
11. Clifton DW. "Tolerated treatment well" may no longer be tolerated. *PT Magazine.* 1995;3(10):24.
12. Abeln SH. Improving functional reporting (utilization review). *PT Magazine.* 1996;4(3):26, 28-30.
13. Stamer MH. *Functional documentation: A process for the physical therapist.* Tucson, AZ: Therapy Skill Builders; 1995.

## Chapter 5

# Rules for Writing in Medical Records

*Mia Erickson, PT, EdD, CHT, ATC*

## Chapter Objectives

Upon completion of this chapter, the reader will be able to:

1. Describe the purpose of the APTA *Guidelines for Physical Therapy Documentation*.
2. Apply basic rules for documenting in medical records.
3. Differentiate between objective and subjective, or unsubstantiated terms written in a note.
4. Describe the importance of using skilled medical language in medical records.
5. List ways to make notes more readable by others.
6. Correctly document late entries and addendums.
7. Correct errors written in a medical record.

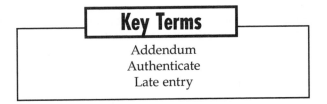

### Key Terms

Addendum
Authenticate
Late entry

# Introduction

The American Physical Therapy Association (APTA) has set forth standardized *Guidelines for Physical Therapy Documentation of Patient/Client Management* (Appendix A) and *Defensible Documentation*.[1] These documents provide documentation guidance for physical therapy professionals across a variety of practice settings.[1] While they are not intended to reflect documentation requirements in all specialty areas, the guidelines can serve as a foundation for developing documentation policies and procedures across a variety of unique and specialized settings.[1] Other authors have also reported specific guidelines for documenting in medical records.[2-10]

From examination to discharge, the physical therapy documentation should reflect: 1) the patient's condition, or pathology, as well as co-morbidities affecting his or her outcome; 2) impairments and functional deficits identified through appropriate, objective tests and measurements; 3) anticipated goals and expected outcomes; 4) interventions provided, including patient education, communication with other disciplines, and specific procedural or therapeutic interventions; and 5) the final outcome, or result of the intervention. It is the position of the APTA that the physical therapy examination, evaluation, diagnosis, and prognosis be documented, dated, and authenticated by the physical therapist (PT) performing the service.[1] Interventions provided by the PT or physical therapist assistant (PTA) should be documented, dated, and authenticated by the PT, or where permissible by law, the PTA, or both.[1] A patient's medical record should be kept in a secured, locked file to meet confidentiality requirements. Following is a list of basic rules for writing in medical records.

# Rules for Writing

- A complete patient record includes: initial examination and evaluations, interim treatment notes and progress reports, regular reassessments, re-examination and re-evaluations when warranted, discharge summaries or notes, physician referral and letters, communication notes, referrals to other health care providers, and any other documentation pertinent to the patient's current condition.

- Document the patient encounter in a timely manner. It is important that documentation is completed as soon after the session as possible. First, the treatment session is fresh in your head, and you are more likely to remember details sooner after the session rather than later. In addition, timely, completed documentation is necessary so that another therapist can treat your patient in the event of your

absence. There are also managerial reasons for timely documentation. These include filing reimbursement claims and sending progress updates to others involved in the patient's care including physicians, case managers, or insurance companies. Clinics and hospitals are likely to have policies in place requiring completion of all patient documentation within a given time frame.

- All entries made in the medical record must be relevant, thorough, accurate, and logical. You should be able to examine your records and have an accurate, detailed depiction of the patient and situation. Any clinician should be able to pick up one of your patient records and treat the patient in the case of your absence.

- Entries must be clear and concise. While it is important to be as concise as possible, you should also be thorough and sufficient in demonstrating the need for skilled services. Never leave out pertinent information for the sake of brevity. As you are learning to write medical records, err on the side of being too lengthy. You can learn to "water down" later after you get more experience and better understand necessary information.

- Be consistent. Use similar types of documentation throughout the patient's episode of care at your facility, ie, forms, SOAP format, flow sheets, etc. This allows reviewers and other health care providers to locate necessary information more easily. Use a similar examination/evaluation form or format for all body parts or diagnoses. Also, use similar forms or writing formats when writing interim notes, re-evaluations, and discharge summaries.

- Use objective language including facts and observations. Avoid making subjective remarks about patients, including anything that cannot be substantiated by objective data. This includes subjective remarks about a patient's response to a treatment (eg, "tolerated treatment well"), the patient's personality, or his or her psychological status ("pt. seemed depressed today"). Also, avoid subjective terms such as "appears" and "seems to be."[11] While you may be trying to provide additional information about the patient, you must be very careful not to make an unsubstantiated judgment for which you are not qualified.[8]

- Write legibly. Third-party payers have been known to deny claims based solely on the fact that they could not read the provider's handwriting. If this is a problem, consider dictating your notes and using a transcription service.

- Use black or blue permanent ink. Ball-point is preferred over felt-tip pens. Erasable ink or pencil should never be used.

- Use scientific, medical terminology. Avoid "non-skilled language" such as "The patient walked..." Use descriptive, functional, and/or medical language instead, such as "Provided gait and transfer training..."

- Describe how you use your unique skills to assist the patient. Provide specific language as to how your special skills and training provided assistance to the patient above and beyond what could be provided by an untrained individual. Description of how your unique and sophisticated skills assisted the patient provides additional insight into the patient's need for skilled services.

*Example 1*:

"Facilitated (R) quadriceps during the swing phase of gait..."

*Example 2*:

"Pt. required min (a) x 1 to manually stabilize (R) knee during stance to prevent hyperextension."

- Use only industry-standard, facility-approved medical terminology, symbols, and abbreviations (Appendix B). Please note that you should not overuse abbreviations. This can become confusing for the reader, especially if he or she is unfamiliar with many of the abbreviations. When reading others' notes, realize some abbreviations have more than one meaning (eg, PT = physical therapist and prothrombin time). In these cases, read the entire note to determine the context of the abbreviation, so that you can interpret it appropriately. Check with your facility regarding acceptable abbreviations and their use.

- Use of first-person is generally not acceptable. Third-person is preferred because the emphasis should be on what the patient can do or does.

*Example*:

*Instead of:* I ambulated the pt. 50' and provided min (a).

*Use*: Pt. ambulated 50' with min (a) x 1

There are times, however when using the first-person is unavoidable. This usually occurs after special situations and you are describing what happened in the narrative format.

- Avoid skipping lines in the record. When writing in a medical record, you should begin your note, starting with the date of service, on the line immediately below the prior entry. Do not skip lines between entries. Furthermore, you should not skip lines in the middle of your notes. Skipping lines could allow someone to come back at a later date and fraudulently add information.

- Use headings. Headings group relevant information together to indicate new sections and to designate important patient information. They often make it easier to read the note and identify necessary information. Examples of appropriate section headings and subheadings can be found in Table 4-1.

- In instances where there is a great deal of data that can easily become confusing to the reader, it is appropriate to use tables, columns, or lists. Tables are valuable when documenting range of motion or strength on several joints such as the hand (Table 5-1).

- Documenting late entries: After completing the documentation for a particular treatment session and placing it in the medical record, you might realize a need to document additional information about the session. You should not rewrite or inappropriately add information to the original note. Instead, complete a late entry or an addendum.

*Late entries*: A chart entry is considered a *late entry* when other health care providers have documented after your original documentation or when enough time has elapsed so that the date on which you are writing the late entry is different from the original documentation. In this case, the entry should be placed in chronological order for the date that it is written and be identified as a "late entry." An explanation for the late entry should also be provided.[2] Sign the late entry as you would any other documentation.

*Addendum*: An addendum is written immediately following the original documentation. In this case, identify the additional information with the heading, "Addendum:" and do not skip a line. Addenda are usually written because you quickly realize you have forgotten to write something that should have been

| | | | AROM | PROM |
|---|---|---|---|---|
| (R) Shoulder | Flexion | | 140° | 155° |
| | Extension | | 10° | 15° |
| | IR | | 50° | 55° |
| | ER | | 45° | 55° |
| (R) Elbow | Flexion | | 140° | 140° |
| | Extension | | -25° | -20° |
| | Supination | | 80° | n/a |
| | Pronation | | 80° | n/a |

Table 5-1

*Sample of Active and Passive Range of Motion Documented in a Table*

included. Sign the addendum as you would your original documentation.

- Correcting errors in medical records: Indicate an error with a single straight line through the text. An individual reading the note should still be able to read what had been written. Initial and date next to the error. Never use correction fluid or erasable ink in a medical record.

*Example*:

The patient ~~ambulated~~ (MLE 2/18/04) transferred with min (a) x 1.

- Date and authenticate all patient records. All physical therapy records should be dated according to the day the services were provided. Authentication is "the process used to verify that an entry into the medical record is complete, accurate, and final. Indications of authentication can include original written signatures and computer 'signatures' on secured electronic record systems only."[1(p703)] Signatures should also include the clinician's full name and designation (PT or PTA).[4] Some states require the PT or PTA provide his or her license number in addition to signature and designation.

- Document reasons for cancelled or missed appointments or treatment sessions, whether initiated by the patient, the PT, the PTA, or another health care provider.

*Example 1*:

In an outpatient clinic, a snowstorm caused your patient to miss two appointments.

Document:

12/19/07—Pt. cancelled appt. 2° to weather. R/S for 12/21.

Sue Brooks, PT

12/21/07—Pt. cancelled 2° to weather. R/S for 12/23.

Sue Brooks, PT

*Example 2*:

On a skilled nursing unit, the nurse asks that you not work with a patient because the physician suspects the patient has a DVT and is awaiting a Doppler.

Document:

12/12/07—Attempted to see Mrs. Smith this a.m. however nursing asked that we hold therapy 2° to possible DVT, awaiting Doppler. Will resume when cleared.

Sue Brooks, PT

- Document all telephone or electronic conversations, such as e-mail, related to patient care. This could include conversations with the patient, the patient's family, the physician, other health care providers, or case managers.

*Example 1*:

You are working with a 24-year-old who was injured in a workplace accident. The patient's case manager for worker's compensation contacts you to determine the patient's status and progress.

Document:

12/22/07—Spoke with pt.'s case manager today and provided update on strength, ROM, and functional status as of re-eval performed on 12/20/07.

Sue Brooks, PT

*Example 2:*

You are working with a patient with Alzheimer's disease who has recently undergone a (R) tibial ORIF 2° to a fracture, and the orthopedic physician ordered "gait training NWB (R) LE." However, 2° to the patient's confusion and inability to follow commands, she is unable to maintain these weight bearing restrictions. You call the physician.

Document:

12/12/07—Called Dr. Jones to make him aware that Mrs. Smith is unable to maintain WB restrictions 2° to confusion & inability to follow commands. Left message. Hold gait training until speaking with physician.

Sue Brooks, PT

- Document verbal orders received or taken from a physician in the following manner:

*Example:*

1/15/07: Verbal order rec'd from Dr. Haines 1/14/07 @ 1:30pm: Please initiate WP to pt's (L) LE.

Sue Brooks, PT

Verbal orders are signed/authenticated by the person taking the order (should be the PT) and signed by the physician giving the verbal order as soon as possible.

- Document any unusual or unexpected situations/results. Some of these situations may also need an incident report completed. Completion of incident reports will be discussed later with legal aspects of documentation. When an unusual event occurs, document the event, the patient's response in objective and measurable terms, your actions or response, and the outcome.

*Example:*

You are working with a 22-year-old female who underwent a right ACL repair. She is performing resisted knee flexion strengthening, feels a "pop" in her knee, and reports an increase in pain from 0/10 to 5/10.

Document:

12/12/07—Pt. was performing (R) knee flexion exercises per ACL protocol & felt a "pop" in her knee. Pain increased from 0/10 to 5/10. Pt. was asked to discontinue her ex. for the day. Rec'd ice to (R) knee for 20'. Called physician & left message for him to call back. After ice, pt. reported a decrease in pain to 0/10 & was able to ambulate without a limp. Will speak with physician about whether he wants to see the pt. or continue per protocol.

Sue Brooks, PT

- When documentation of patient care requires more than one page, make sure subsequent or additional pages include the patient's name, patient or chart number, and the date. Transition the information by writing a statement like:

"(Cont. next page—Sue Brooks, PT)"

Then, on the next page write: "(Cont. from previous)"

# Review Questions

1.  What components of patient care should be reflected in physical therapy documentation?

2.  What is the purpose of the APTA's *Guidelines for Physical Therapy Documentation of Patient/Client Management* and *Defensible Documentation?*

3.  Give one example of how documentation from examination to discharge can be consistent.

4.  Give one example of a statement that would be considered "unsubstantiated" or an unqualified judgment of a patient.

5.  What ink colors are most appropriate for writing in medical records?

6.  What is the purpose of using medical language and terms describing your unique contribution to assisting the patient?

7.  How much time should elapse between treating the patient and documenting the encounter?

8.  What does the term "authenticate" mean?

9.  What factors differentiate a "late entry" from an "addendum?"

10.  Examine your state's physical therapy practice act.
    a. Are there regulations or requirements for documenting physical therapy? If so, what are they?
    b. Are there regulations or requirements for PTs that are different for PTAs? If so, what are they?
    c. Are PTAs required to have notes co-signed by a PT? How does this vary, or differ dependent on practice setting?
    d. How do documentation regulations or requirements in your state's practice act differ from the Model Practice Act issued by the Federation of State Boards of Physical Therapy (www.fsbpt.org)?

# Application Exercises

I. For the following entries, indicate ones that are inappropriate by writing an "I" next to the item. Describe why they are inappropriate.

_____ The patient walked 50'.

_____ This patient requires skilled services.

_____ Pt. stated that she enjoys coming to PT.

_____ Pt. c/o pain in the (L) knee following exercise after last visit.

_____ AROM: (R) shoulder flexion 160° abduction 120°

_____ Pt. performed QS, GS, and SLRs.

_____ Pt. walked around the PT gym 2x

_____ Pt. reported compliance with his HEP and ↑ AROM.

_____ Pt. is demonstrating excessive hip abduction with his prosthesis during ambulation

_____ Gait: 100' with hemi-walker with min (a) x 1 for trunk support & min (a) x 1 for advancing the (L) LE

_____ Transfers: Bed → chair with min (a) x 1 2° to poor balance

_____ Ther Ex: Performed 20 repetitions all exercises

_____ Bed Mobility: Rolls supine → SL with min (a) x 1

_____ HEP: Instructed the pt. in a HEP to be performed tid.

_____ The pt. reported to PT today in a wheelchair with his leg on an elevated leg rest, which is the same way he was transported to PT all week.

II. Write the following information in a more clear, concise manner, as it would appear in the medical record.

1. The patient walked 75 feet in the hallway of the hospital with the therapist lightly touching her back (often referred to as contact guard assist, or CGA). She used a front-wheeled walker.

2. The patient's strength was 3/5 for the right biceps and 4/5 for the right triceps.

3. Upon arrival to therapy, the patient told you that she has been doing her HEP without any problems and really feels like her ability to reach into an overhead cupboard has improved.

4. The patient said that her pain was 3/10 on a pain scale.

5. The patient demonstrated the following ROM measurements: active ROM for the right elbow was 130° flexion and 10° of hyperextension.

6. (L) Knee active ROM was 100° flexion and lacking 10° of extension.

7. The patient propelled his wheelchair around the hospital 250', outside on the sidewalk 50', and up and down several ramps with you providing verbal reminders on trunk positioning for going up and down the ramp.

8. The patient walked 50 feet using the wide-based quad cane and the AFO on the right ankle. She needed minimal assistance to swing the right leg to prevent getting her toes caught on the floor. The patient was able to put her ankle-foot orthosis on and remove it independently. She was also able to check her skin for any irritated areas after she removed it.

9. You instructed the patient to perform 10 repetitions of each exercise as part of her home exercise program. The exercises included ankle pumps, quadriceps setting, short arc quadriceps strengthening from 45° to 0, and heel slides.

10. During a busy morning in the hospital, you were working with a patient who told you that she was going to be discharged and wanted home health services, primarily PT. After writing the note and completing your morning treatment sessions, you realize that you did not document your patient's desire for home PT. What should you do? How you would document this entry into the chart? Where should this information be placed?

11. After documenting a patient's ROM, you realize that you made an error. It should have been 125°, not 152°. Demonstrate below how to correct this mistake if you find it immediately.

AROM: shoulder flexion 152°

III. Organize the following subjective and objective information so that it is clear and concise, suitable for entry into the medical record.

1. Mr. Jones comes in to the clinic today and tells you that his fingers became swollen and that he has had pain at a level of 7 out of 10 since the last treatment session. He goes on to say that he has not been able to perform any of the ROM exercises you gave him because of the incredible amount of pain he has been having. He said that he has changed his post-operative dressing once a day and he has had a little bit

of red drainage on the bandages. He also said that he is having trouble eating and shaving due to the swelling and stiffness in the joints.

2. You enter Mrs. Smith's hospital room and ask her if she is ready for treatment. She agrees and tells you that she wants to be ready for walking down the aisle at her grandson's wedding with her walker. She said that her right knee pain is not as bad as it was yesterday, and she thinks that she is able to bend it more as well. She goes on to say that she has performed the ROM exercises twice already this morning, and she is working on trying to get her knee to bend as much as she can. She asks if she can begin using a cane soon.

3. You are assigned an inpatient who had a right cerebral vascular accident 3 weeks ago. She is demonstrating confusion and slurred speech, but her daughter is usually present during the sessions. Upon entering the patient's room, you notice the daughter is not present. As you work with the patient, she tells you that last night she fell in the bathroom. She also tells you that she is afraid to get out of bed because of her fear of falling again. It was difficult for you to understand the patient due to the slurring. You also understand the patient to say that her left shoulder is sore. Toward the end of the session, her daughter returns and you comment to the daughter about the patient's fall the previous night. The daughter tells you that there wasn't a fall and that she had been there with her mother all night.

4. While treating a patient during a home health visit, the patient's son tells you that his mother (the patient) has been up all night due to left hip pain. He also tells you that he is having trouble getting his mother to walk in the house with him due to pain and fear of making her hip hurt more than it already is. He also says that he has trouble performing the ROM exercises that you showed him during the last session. The patient tells you that she feels like her hip is going to give out when she stands on it due to the pain.

5. AROM measurements for the (R) UE and LE are as follows: knee flexion 100°, extension 5° hip abduction 20° hip flexion 100°, ankle PF 20°, elbow AROM 10-100, shoulder flexion 100°, shoulder abduction 100°, hip IR 20°, ankle DF 5°, shoulder ER 60° and IR 45°

6. The patient walked with the therapist at his side (but not touching him) for 100 feet, twice; vitals signs before exercise were blood pressure 125/85, 15 for respirations and 77 for heart rate. Vitals after were 135/85 for blood pressure, 17 for respirations, and 87 for heart rate. The patient performed ankle pumping, elbow flexion, shoulder flexion, knee extension for 10 repetitions before and after ambulation.

7. Girth at the right knee medial joint line was 34 cm, 2 inches above was 38 cm, 4 inches above was 42 cm, and 4 inches below was 35.5 cm. Active knee flexion was 120°. The patient lacked 20° of active extension in the knee. Hip and ankle active ROM were within normal limits. Strength for the quad muscle was 3-/5, and for the hamstring was 3-/5. All measurements for (R) LE. The patient walks independently with crutches, weight bearing as much as he can tolerate on the involved extremity.

8. You are working with a patient in an outpatient clinic with a diagnosis of bicipital tendonitis. She tells you that she has been working on the home exercises and overall her arm is feeling much better. She reports pain to be 3/10 on a verbal pain scale. She says that she has trouble reaching into overhead cabinets and shelves. Her treatment consisted of phonophoresis over the anterior shoulder for 8 minutes, 50% duty cycle with the intensity set at 1.5 w/cm². This was followed by gentle active ROM exercises with a wand for flexion and external rotation, active scapular retraction and protraction, prone horizontal abduction, and external rotation with yellow theraband for 2 sets of 10 repetitions. She also received manual stretching for flexion internal rotation, and external rotation (performed by you). The total exercise session lasted 30 minutes. The treatment concluded with ice for 15 minutes.

9. You are working with a patient 3 days status post right total knee replacement in the PT gym. She transfers to and from the mat with you providing 25% assistance. She transferred sit to and from supine with you performing 50% assistance due to her inability to lift the right leg onto the mat table. She performed 2 sets of 10 repetitions of the total knee exercises and ambulated 50 feet, twice with a standard walker, only putting 50% of her body weight on the involved extremity. She received ice for 15 minutes to her knee.

## Identifying Documentation Errors

Directions: List problems with the following initial exam/evaluation reports.

## Example 1

**Therapist**: John Smith, PT
**Physician**: Dr. Harris
**Date**: November 7, 2005
**Diagnosis**: s/p (R) rotator cuff repair and acromioplasty
**ICD-9**: 840.4

Functional Impairments: Patient is limited in any activity requiring overhead or active movement of the (R) UE.

Date of onset: Patient fell and injured (R) shoulder on October 2, 2005. Surgery was November 1, 2005.

Next MD Appt: December 7, 2005

Diagnostic tests: MRI. See attached report

History/Relevant subjective: Patient fell on October 2, 2005 landing on (R) UE. After fall, he complained of significant pain and sought medical attention. MRI revealed partial thickness tear of rotator cuff. Underwent repair to (R) rotator cuff by Dr. Harris on November 1, 2005. Patient reports point tenderness along the spine of the scapula and is limiting him from performing his ADLs. Patient has not been sleeping well and reports pain at 8/10 on the pain scale. Patient has difficulty raising his arm overhead due to pain however pain decreases when arm is placed on his stomach. Patient would like to improve independence in ADLs without pain and perform home management tasks.

Objective: Asymetrical arm movement during gait. AROM: flexion 30°, abduction 90°, IR 80°, ER 15°. PROM: flexion 60°, abduction 100°, IR 70°, ER 20°. Resistive testing found flexion, abduction and ER weak and painful. Electrodes placed over the (R) shoulder for premod e-stim 80-150 x 20 minutes with ice.

Assessment: s/p (R) rotator cuff repair and acromioplasty

STGs:
Decrease pain from 6/10 to 4/10 within 2-3 weeks
Increase PROM 10-20° in flexion, abduction, and ER

Discharge Goals:
Independently perform ADLs within 6-8 weeks
Decrease complaints of pain to 0/10 within 6-8 weeks
Obtain functional ROM within 6-8 weeks

Rehab Potential: Good

Interventions to be used: Modalities, ultrasound, electric stimulation, laser. Manual therapy, PROM, stretching and joint mobilizations. Therapeutic exercises and activities will be performed per protocol.

Frequency and Duration of Treatment: 2-3 times per week for 8-12 weeks at discretion of physician to increase strength of glenohumeral and scapular muscles, ROM, and decrease pain.

## Example 2

**Date**: March 1, 2005

**Subjective/History**: Pt. c/o mild, achy pain in the upper and lower thoracic region. Pain is noted with sitting, especially with a slumped posture. Pt. is RHD. Pt. is involved with youth basketball.

**Objective**: Standing Posture: Right thoracic convexity and left lumbar convexity. Displays kypholordotic curvature. Right rib hump. PSIS and iliac crests are equal heights bil. Right foot more pronated than left. AROM with flexion: pt. veers to the right with full ROM. Displays full extension with a hinge point at L4-L5. Bil. side flexion and rotation are full. Pt. hamstrings are minimally tight. Quadriceps are not tight. Both hip abductors and adductors are 3-/5. Paraspinals are 3/5 with difficulty. Pt. rx today consists of initial evaluation and therapeutic exercise of shoulder ER, horizontal abduction, & D2 flexion/extension pattern with yellow theraband. Pt. performed 1 set of 10 reps. HEP consists of 10 x 3 sets 2-3x/day of each exercise. Pt. educated on proper posture and the use of a lumbar roll for correct posture. Pt's mother present for treatment session.

**Assessment**: 14 y.o. female with scoliosis. Referred by CRNP after x-rays. Postural dysfunction and weakness.

STGs: Within 1-2 weeks, the pt. will:
Independence in HEP
Improve strength to 4/5 on convex side
Improve flexibility on concave side

Discharge goals: Within 3-4 weeks, the pt. will:
1. be independent with a HEP, maintenance, and prevention programs
2. have a good understanding of the importance of correct, erect posture, and maintaining exercise following therapy
3. be independent with lumbar stabilization techniques and understand the importance of neutral pelvis

**Plan**: See pt. in clinic 2x/wk x 4 wks. For therapeutic exercise, postural education, lumbar stabilization training, neuromuscular re-education, manual therapy, and pt. education.
Suzy Smith, PT

## Example 3

**Date**: March 1, 2005

**History**: 15 y.o. female with (B) Achilles tendon pain starting last August. PMH: (B) patellofemoral pain syndrome. Referred by physician last week for PT 3x/wk x 1month with dx of (B) equines. No meds. C/C: Increased pain in (B) Achilles with repetitive jumping and after sports. Home situation: Lives with her parents and attends school. Pt.'s goal to return to jumping pain free and be ready for softball season. Pain level 3/10 right and 4/10 on left.

**O**: AROM:

|  | Right | Left |
|---|---|---|
| DF | 2° | 6° |
| PF | WNL | WNL |
| Ev | WNL | WNL |

| Strength: | | |
|---|---|---|
| DF | 5/5 | 5/5 |
| PF | 5/5 | 5/5 |
| Inv | 5/5 | 5/5 |
| Ev | 5/5 | 5/5 |

*(continued)*

## Example 3, continued

Girth:         1-1/2′  32-1/2cm    33-1/4cm
               from
               calcaneus

Edema:              (-)             (-)
Tenderness:         (-)             (-)
Sensation:          Intact          Intact
                    to light        to light
                    touch           touch

<u>Today's Tx</u>: <u>Pt. Education</u>-condition and what we will be doing in therapy to help correct it
<u>Ther Exercise</u>-Gastroc-soleus stretching 3x30 seconds each; supination and pronation in standing to fatigue; towel curls

<u>PT Diagnosis</u>: Practice Pattern 4F Impaired joint mobility, motor function, muscle performance, and range of motion associated with localized inflammation

**A**: 15 y.o. female c/o (B) Achilles pain after activity such as jumping and recreational activities

Problem list:
1. Unable to run
2. Unable to jump
3. Unable to participate in recreational activities
4. Pain level 3/10 right; 4/10 left

STGs: In 2 weeks, pt. will
1. Decrease pain after activity to 2/10
2. Be able to tolerate fast-paced walking x 20 min.
3. Increase DF to 8° right and 10° left

Discharge goals: In 4 weeks, the pt. will:
1. Pain free in (B) Achilles
2. Return to normal recreational activities without c/o pain
3. ROM WNL
4. Independent and complaint with HEP

Plan: See pt. 3x/wk x 2 weeks for:
1. Functional training
2. Flexibility
3. HEP

Joe Thompson, PT

---

## Example 4

*Physical Therapy Report*

**Date**: 4/5/05

**S**: 67 y.o. male brought to ER 4/2/05 with unrelenting chest pain and tightness. Admitting dx: MI. Now 1 day s/p CABG x3. No current complaints. Lives in two-story home with wife, bedroom on second floor with 1 flight of steps and a handrail on the right. Retired but enjoys active lifestyle including farming. Pt.'s goal to return to previous active lifestyle.

**O**: From the chart: Height: 6'2" Weight: 345#. BP 135/75, HR 78, RR 10. Transferred out of bed to chair with mod assist x 2. Ambulation not assessed at this time secondary to protocol. Performed 10 reps CABG post-op exercise.

**A**: 1 day s/p CABG x3. Problems: limited mobility STGs: In two days pt. will ambulate in the hallway with supervision and transfer in/out of bed with min assist. Discharge goals: In 5-7 days pt. will ambulate 150-200' with supervision and transfer independently.

**P**: See pt. bid for CABG protocol.

John Smith, PT

---

# References

1. American Physical Therapy Association. *The Guide to Physical Therapist Practice*. Alexandria, VA: APTA; 2001.

2. Abeln SH. Liability awareness. Reporting risk check-up. *PT Magazine*. 1997;5(10):38-42.

3. Arriaga R. Liability awareness. Stories from the front: documentation and clinical decision making: a real-life scenario illustrates some basic risk-management principles. *PT Magazine*. 2002;10(5):46-9.

4. Goode N. The reliable resource: physical therapy documentation. *PT Magazine*. 1999;7(9):30-1.

5. Inaba M, Jones SL. Medical documentation for third-party payers. *Phys Ther*. 1977;57(7):791-4.

6. Redgate N, Foto M. Pay by the rules: avoid Medicare audits and reduce payment denials with a sound strategy and proper documentation. *Physical Therapy Products*. 2003;October/November:28-30.

7. Scholey ME. Documentation: a means of professional development... in physiotherapy. *Physiotherapy*. 1985;71(6):276-8.

8. Schunk CR. Liability awareness. Advice for the new physical therapist: here are some keys to avoiding risk once you've made the transition from student to practitioner. *PT Magazine*. 2001;9(11):24-26.

9. White JA. Managing care. Documentation: making it meaningful. *Physical Therapy Case Reports*. 2000;3(2):78-9.

10. Lewis DK. Do the write thing: document everything. *PT Magazine*. 2002;10(7):30-34.

11. Clifton DW. "Tolerated treatment well" may no longer be tolerated. *PT Magazine*. 1995;3(10):24.

## Chapter 6

# Recording Subjective Information

*Rebecca McKnight, PT, MS*

## Chapter Objectives

Upon completion of this chapter, the reader will be able to:

1. List sources of information for subjective (history) data.
2. Identify types of data that should be recorded in the subjective portion of a SOAP note.
3. Discuss how subjective data is used to inform the clinical decision-making process.
4. Discuss how subjective data should correlate with information in the objective, assessment, and plan portions of a SOAP note.
5. Analyze given information and determine additional subjective data that should be gathered.
6. Arrange data collected from history-taking into a logically sequenced subjective note.
7. Discuss how the physical therapist assistant will use the subjective information found in an initial evaluative note.

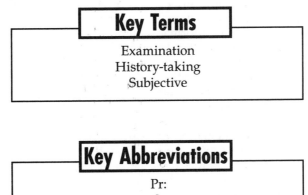

### Key Terms

Examination
History-taking
Subjective

### Key Abbreviations

Pr:
S:

| Table 6-1 *Where the Elements of the Patient/Client Management Model Can Be Found in a SOAP Note* | |
|---|---|
| *Patient/Client Management Model* | *SOAP Evaluative Note* |
| **Examination** | |
| • History | Problem (Pr:) Subjective (S:) |
| • Systems Review<br>• Tests and Measurements | Objective (O:) |
| **Evaluation**<br>**Diagnosis**<br>**Prognosis** | Assessment (A:) |
| **Intervention** | Plan (P:) |

## Introduction

Every day, all across America, physical therapy care is being initiated. Individuals with a variety of medical conditions, impairments, functional limitations, and disabilities are turning to physical therapists (PTs) to help them manage their conditions and meet their physical goals. The importance of documentation as a part of the physical therapy process cannot be over-emphasized. Although many times documentation is seen as "paperwork" or simply recording activities that occur, documentation has a vital role in the clinical decision-making process and in care delivery.

While documentation is necessary across the entire spectrum of physical therapy care, documentation of the initiation of physical therapy services holds a unique and important role. It is within this initial evaluation that the therapist is able to capture and document pertinent information that demonstrates the patient's concerns as well as vital patient information. Documentation of the initial evaluation should also clearly detail the physical therapy plan of care, including the expected outcomes and intervention strategies to be used. It is upon this plan of care that future physical therapy visits will be based.

In order to be able to make appropriate decisions about the patient's diagnosis and determine the prognosis and intervention plan, the therapist must first gather information. This gathering of data is referred to in *The Guide to Physical Therapist Practice* as the *examination*. The examination has three components: 1) history-taking, 2) systems review, and 3) tests and measures.[1(p34)] Writing this information down (documenting) helps the therapist gain a clearer picture of the patient's status and provides a framework on which comparisons and clinical decision-making can occur (Table 6-1).

## What Is Subjective Information?

Subjective data correlates with the history-taking component of the examination as outlined in The *Guide to Physical Therapist Practice*. The *Guide* defines this process as "a systematic gathering of data from both the past and the present–related to why the patient/client is seeking the services of the physical therapist"[1(p34)] (Figure 6-1). Subjective data is information that the therapist gleans through ways other than through direct observation. During the history-taking component of the examination, the PT will include data gathered from the medical record, the patient, and/or the patient's family or caregiver. Collection of the subjective information is an essential part of the examination and evaluation process. Subjective information gathered from the patient is used by the PT to form a clear picture of what the patient knows and understands about his or her condition and its impact on his or her functional status and roles.

Webster's dictionary defines subjective as "characteristic of or belonging to reality as perceived rather than as independent of mind", "peculiar to a particular individual", "modified or affected by personal views, experience, or background" and "lacking in reality or substance."[2] These definitions imply that subjective information may be lacking in validity or reliability due to the personal perspectives attained. As PTs, we need to keep in mind that subjective data gathered from the patient does in fact carry that individual's personal perspective, and this perspective should be a central component of the clinical decision-making process.[3]

### Where Does It Come From?

In most cases, subjective information is data gathered from the patient through direct and specific

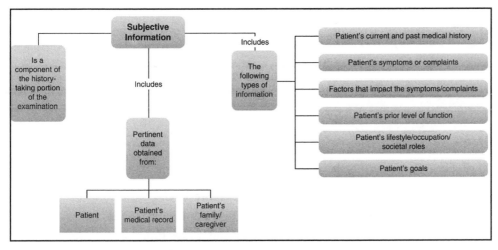

**Figure 6-1.** Subjective information.

questioning. Individuals who are in close relationships with the patient may also be able to provide direct information about the patient's condition and functional status. The patient's family or caregiver can provide additional information and alternate perspectives that can help form a more comprehensive view of the patient's status. In cases where the patient has cognitive or communicative limitations and where no medical records exist, the subjective information may come entirely from the family or caregiver. In these situations, the therapist should identify the individual who has the closest contact with the patient. This person will likely be the individual who can provide the clearest picture of the patient's functional abilities and limitations.

In addition, subjective data can be gleaned from the patient's medical record, when it is available. The medical record can be a rich source of data. Whenever possible, verify information found in the medical record directly with the patient or patient's family/caregiver. Inconsistencies between the medical record and the patient's reports should be investigated. Errors in medical reporting do occur and clinical decision-making based upon false information can lead to negative results. Alternatively, the inconsistency could demonstrate the patient's flawed understanding of the problem or perhaps could illuminate dishonest or deceptive patient motives. These types of problems should be rectified in order for appropriate expectations and realistic outcomes to be determined.

## What Type of Information Is It?

Subjective information includes data that provides insight into the patient's condition and its impact on the patient's functional mobility and activity participation. The therapist should glean all information available regarding the medical diagnosis, impairments in body functions, functional limitations, and activity restrictions related to the current condition. This information will also help the PT discern the patient's affective response to these issues. The primary focus of subjective information should be the patient's current condition.

However, existing co-morbidities, other medical or physical restrictions, as well as past medical or physical conditions must be identified and documented. Contextual factors (environment or personal) that impact the patient's daily life should also be determined and included in the documentation of subjective data. Examples of contextual factors to document include: 1) characteristics of the environment(s) in which the patient functions (home, work, community), 2) availability of support systems (family, societal), and 3) patient attitudes and attitudes of the patient's support network (family, friends, caregivers).

Table 6-2 provides a list of types of data that may be generated during the "history-taking" process.[1] Specific questions to ask will be determined by the physical therapist as part of the clinical decision-making process.

### General Demographics

General demographic information, ie, age, sex, race/ethnicity, primary language and level of education, help to provide a global picture of the patient. This information can assist in identification of risk factors and will be useful in the evaluation process when determining the diagnosis, prognosis, and plan of care.

### Current Conditions/Chief Complaints

Clearly identifying the patient's primary complaint(s) is a natural starting point for most clinicians. This provides the clinician with a foundation for clinical decision-making and provides the patient with the opportunity to share his/her concerns. This interchange should also facilitate the development of trust between the patient and the practitioner —an important factor in rehabilitation. The therapist should ask for detailed information in order to

| Table 6-2 |
| --- |
| *Subjective Types of Data* |

General Demographics
- Age
- Sex
- Race/ethnicity
- Primary language
- Education

Current Conditions/Chief Complaints
- Concerns that led the patient to seek the services of a physical therapist
- Current therapeutic interventions
- Mechanisms of injury or disease, including date of onset and course of events
- Onset and pattern of symptoms
- Pt./client, family, sig. other, and caregiver expectations and goals
- Pt./client, family, sig. other, and caregiver perceptions of pt's emotional response to the current situation
- Previous occurrence of the same complaints/symptoms
- Prior therapeutic interventions

Medical/Surgical Hx
- Cardiovascular
- Endocrine/metabolic
- Gastrointestinal
- Genitourinary
- Gynecological
- Integumentary
- Musculoskeletal
- Neuromuscular
- Obstetrical
- Prior hospitalizations, surgeries, and preexisting medical and other health-related conditions
- Psychological
- Pulmonary

Medications
- For current condition
- Previously taken for current condition
- For other conditions

Other Clinical Tests
- Lab and diagnostic test

- Review of available records
  - Medical
  - Education
  - Surgical
- Review of other clinical findings
  - Nutrition
  - Hydration

Functional Status and Activity Level
- Current and prior functional status in self-care and home management
  - ADL
  - IADL
- Current and prior functional status in:
  - work (job/school/play)
  - Community
  - Leisure

Social History
- Cultural beliefs and behaviors
- Family and caregiver resources
- Social interactions, social activities and support systems

Living Environment
- Devices and equipment
- Living environment and community characteristics
- Projected discharge destinations

General Health Status
- General health perception
- Physical function
  - Mobility
  - Sleep patterns
- Psychological function
  - Memory
  - Reasoning ability
  - Depression
  - Anxiety
- Role function
  - Community
  - Leisure
  - Social
  - Work

| Table 6-2, continued | |
|---|---|
| *Subjective Types of Data* | |

| | |
|---|---|
| • Social function | Family History |
|    – Social activity |   • Family health risks |
|    – Social interaction | Employment/Work |
|    – Social support |   • Current and prior work |
| Social/Health Habits (Past & Current) |    – Job |
|   • Behavioral health risks |    – School |
|    – Smoking |    – Play |
|    – Drug abuse |   • Community |
|   • Level of physical fitness |   • Leisure |
| Growth & Development | |
|   • Developmental hx | Compiled from figure 2 in *The Guide to Physical Therapist Practice.*[1] |
|   • Hand dominance | |

obtain a clear picture of the patient's complaints and concerns. Details of the mechanism of injury or disease, including date of onset, course of events that lead up to the current condition, onset and pattern of symptoms and any previous occurrence of the same complaints/symptoms provide vital information that assists the therapist in the diagnostic process. During the history-taking, or interview process, the therapist should be attentive and monitor for verbal remarks and non-verbal signs that demonstrate patient's (family member/caregiver's) perceptions of the patient's current status. It is important to remember that the patient's perspective may conflict with the reality of the situation and can have a significant impact on his or her therapy goals and outcomes.

The therapist should ascertain all prior and current therapeutic interventions for any of the patient's current conditions and their effectiveness. This includes interventions provided in traditional medical settings, as well as any alternative medicine or home remedy solutions the patient has used. Awareness of the level of effectiveness of prior and current interventions will provide the therapist with information that is useful in determining the plan of care. This information can also help in distinguishing treatment effects of physical therapy interventions versus other interventions the patient is receiving (or has received) for the same condition.

As part of gathering data related to the patient's condition, the patient's expectations and goals must be considered and documented. Inadequate understanding or appreciation for the patient's goals could lead to the therapist setting goals that the patient doesn't buy into. The patient's level of participation in the therapy process is closely tied to how well the established goals and expected outcomes mirror the patient's personal goals for therapy.

## Medical/Surgical History

Whenever possible, information regarding the patient's medical and surgical history should be obtained from the medical record. The medical record will provide details that the patient is often unable to recall or may not understand. These details can assist the therapist in gaining a full picture of the patient's condition. For example, a patient might report that the total knee replacement surgery was described by the surgeon as "difficult". Upon review of the surgical report, the therapist can identify details of the surgical procedure that can guide the therapist in determining specific intervention strategies and in setting realistic goals/outcome expectations. As data is collected, any prior medical/surgical procedures including procedures affecting the cardiovascular, endocrine/metabolic, gastrointestinal, genitourinary, gynecological, integumentary, musculoskeletal, neuromuscular, obstetrical, psychological, and pulmonary systems should be noted. Often during the initial examination/evaluation process some information may not appear to be relevant to the patient's current condition. However, it is not uncommon that during the course of an episode of care, the patient's past medical or surgical history sheds significant light on the patient's problems and progress in physical therapy.

When the medical record is not readily available (such as in the outpatient clinic setting), the patient or patient's caregiver should be encouraged to share as much medical information as possible. In these situations, it may sometimes be necessary to request copies of the patient's record so that the therapist will be able to gain an adequate understanding of the patient's condition in order to formulate a safe and effective intervention plan.

## Medications

The importance of considering the pharmacologic management of the patient receiving physical therapy has grown in recent years as the profession has matured. As an autonomous practitioner, it is imperative that the PT remembers to take into account the impact of medications on the patient's status. Documentation of medications that are currently being and have previously been used for the current condition as well as the effectiveness of the medication for its stated purpose(s) should occur. For example, the PT might record the patient's reports of pain relief from the use of current or previous pain medications.

Any current medications prescribed for other conditions should also be documented. Identification of medications the patient is using is crucial in evaluation and intervention planning. The therapist should consider the impact of the medications on the patient's current condition (will it help or hinder the healing process?). It is often necessary for the therapist to consult with the physician regarding medication adjustments so that the patient will be able to effectively participate in physical therapy and so the patient's goals can be achieved. For example, when working with a patient who has Parkinson's disease, the PT can provide information about the patient's mobility status that will assist the physician in determining dosage levels and medication scheduling.

Understanding the side effects of pharmacologic agents can also provide insight into the patient's responses to activity or exercise. For example, patients who are utilizing beta blockers for various cardiopulmonary disorders might experience abnormal blood pressure responses to exercise. It is important for the therapist to be prepared for this response and be careful to note other factors that may influence the patient's response to physical activity.

## Other Clinical Tests

Equally important to consider during the examination and evaluation are results of lab and diagnostic tests. Lab results can provide a unique view into the patient's status. For example, a patient who is in the acute recovery stage after an orthopedic surgery may have low hemoglobin and hematocrit (H&H) values. Upon considering the total picture of the patient, the therapist may choose to limit the intervention activities to only bedside activities. The therapist should review available medical and surgical records and document any information that is pertinent to the physical therapy process, such as information about the patient's nutritional status or hydration level. Again, this information can provide a valuable perspective into the patient's responses during the physical therapy interventions.

## Functional Status and Activity Level

To help guide the process of determining future outcomes, the patient's current and prior functional status in self-care and home management should be considered and documented. Recording the patient's prior and current functional status with activities of daily living (ADLs), such as the patient's ability to maneuver in and out of bed or ambulate around the house, will provide information regarding how the disease or injury has affected the patient's day-to-day life. Also important to consider and document is the patient's prior and current functional status in instrumental activities of daily living (IADL), such as activities at work (including job/school/play), activities in the community (such as involvement in religious organizations or volunteer groups), and leisure activities (such as gardening or canoeing). Again, this provides information as to how the disease or injury has affected the patient's day-to-day life and participation in society. It may also provide the therapist with a better understanding of the patient's potential and provide information from which the therapist can draw to help motivate the patient during the intervention process. The therapist should consider these activities and incorporate them into the plan of care when formulating the therapy goals and intervention strategies.

## Social History

The patient's social history further provides a picture of contextual factors that can impact an individual's functioning in society. This information can be used to determine appropriate goals for the patient as well as guide the therapist in locating resources to support the patient during and after the episode of care. The therapist should gather information about family and caregiver resources, cultural beliefs and behaviors, the patient's social interactions, social activities, and support systems. The World Health Organization's *International Classification of Functioning, Disability and Health* (ICF) model currently is designed to take the contextual factors of social systems into account when classifying the patient's functional status. "Disability is characterized as the outcome or result of a complex relationship between an individual's health condition and personal factors, and of the external factors that represent the circumstances in which the individual lives. Because of this relationship, different environments may have a very different impact on the same individual with a given health condition."[4(p17)] It is imperative that the PT take these contextual factors into consideration when designing the plan of care. To neglect to do so may result in a failure to reach the expected outcomes.[3]

## Living Environment

From the initial evaluation, the therapist should consider the patient's projected discharge destination. This should include identification of the patient's current living environment and characteristics as well as any devices and equipment the patient already owns. When there is a question as to whether the patient will be able to return to his or her current living environment, additional inquiry should be made into alternate living arrangements that are available. For example, consider a 98-year-old female who has sustained a hip fracture and is to maintain toe-touch weight bearing precautions during gait. This patient may not be able to return to living independently in her single-wide trailer in a rural area immediately. However, during the history-taking process, the PT learns that the patient does have the option of residing with her granddaughter in a ranch-style home where family will be available to provide assistance during her recovery.

## General Health Status

Documentation of the patient's general health status should include the patient's perception of his or her general health, general physical function (mobility, sleep patterns), psychological function (memory, reasoning ability, depression, anxiety), role function in the community (leisure, social, work), and social function (social activities, social interaction, social support). This can be accomplished through direct questioning or through a health-related quality of life questionnaire. Identification of the patient's general health status will assist the therapist in determining appropriate goals and outcome expectations. Factors that may indicate the need for referral to another health care provider can also be determined through a review of the patient's general health status. For example, during the interview process, a patient may reveal a history of issues with anxiety and what the patient describes as "panic attacks." If the patient indicates he or she has not sought any assistance for these issues, the PT could inform the patient of resources available, such as the primary medical physician or a psychologist, for future assessment of the patient's psychological health.

## Social/Health Habits (Past and Current)

Lifestyle habits, whether past or current, including behavioral health risks habits such as smoking or drug use/abuse and physical fitness habits, are important to identify. Habits such as smoking can impact healing time and therefore may influence the time to achieve the ultimate outcome (timeline) and the patient's progress during the interventions. The patient's general physical fitness habits should also be taken into account. For example, a patient who reports habits of frequent heavy physical fitness activities may require additional education on the detrimental effects that can occur if inappropriate stresses are placed upon healing tissues. This information will also guide the therapist in goal setting. A patient who is accustomed to significant physical exertion will likely have more strenuous outcome expectations than the expectations of a patient who has a sedentary lifestyle.

## Growth and Development

Issues related to growth and development should always be considered when dealing with the pediatric client. Gathering data related to the child's developmental history will provide valuable information that will guide the therapist's evaluation process, including selecting appropriate tests and measures to use during the objective data collection, determining the diagnosis and prognosis, and structuring the intervention plan. Growth and developmental history should also be documented when evaluating adults with a prior medical history that includes a developmental disorder.

Documentation of hand dominance is also important at times. This information can impact outcome expectations and intervention strategies. For example, a patient who has a brachial plexus injury resulting in a non-functioning right extremity may have differing expectations if the injury occurred in the dominant extremity versus the non-dominant extremity.

## Family History

Family health risks should be identified and are used as a screening mechanism to be viewed along with other subjective and objective data. Identification of health risks may illuminate a need for referral to another health care provider. For example, a 40-year-old female is seeking physical therapy services for management of her headaches. During the history-taking portion of the examination process, the patient divulges that both her mother and her maternal grandmother had "uncontrolled blood pressure" and that her maternal grandmother had a mild stroke and died from an aortic aneurysm. This information combined with the patient's borderline hypertensive blood pressure reading would alert the therapist to recommend that the patient seek attention from her physician.

## Employment/Work

Information should be gathered regarding the patient's current and prior work status. Information regarding current work status will provide the therapist with information to guide establishment of goals and determination of appropriate and efficient intervention strategies. For individuals who are retired or disabled and are no longer employed, information about prior work status can help the therapist gain a better perspective of the patient's physical conditioning and general health. This information can also provide tips for activities the therapist can use when structuring interventions to help motivate the patient.

*The Guide to Physical Therapist Practice* also includes participation in school or play activities in this category to address issues for pediatric clients and adults whose primary role, or "job" is as a student. Consideration of these environments and the activities in which the patient normally participates should be included in the documentation.

# Importance of Documenting Subjective Information

Clinical decision-making should flow from a well-documented clinical examination that creates a picture of the patient, including the patient's impairments in body structure and function, functional activities and participation (and any limitations of these), and the contextual factors (environmental and personal) that impact the patient. Subjective information is required to develop this detailed view of the patient. During the history-taking portion of the examination process, the therapist will be developing a clinical hypothesis regarding the patient's problem(s) and will begin to make determinations of specific tests and measures to perform. Subjective information will be used in conjunction with the objective data obtained during the tests and measures portion of the examination in order to support the PT's evaluation of the patient. The diagnosis, prognosis, outcome expectations, and interventions should be supported by the subjective (as well as the objective) data obtained.

In addition to gathering data for determination of a diagnosis and prognosis, the subjective information can provide a view into the psychosocial issues and contextual factors that influence the patient's functioning and participation. The PT should take all these factors into consideration when designing a plan of care. Therefore, two different patients with the same diagnosis can likely have two very different intervention plans due to factors such as age, goals, expectations, and social dynamics among others.

# How to Document Subjective Information

Every documentation entry made should begin with the patient's identification information such as the patient's name, any record or patient number, and the date. For an initial examination and evaluation, the reason(s) for referral and the referral source (eg, physician name or self-referral) should also be included. Often at the beginning of a SOAP note, there is a "Problem" (Pr:) section that provides or lists the patient's primary problem(s). The problem can be stated as the medical or referring diagnosis, the physical therapy diagnosis, the impairment(s) of body structures or functions, or activity and participation restrictions (functional limitations) (Example 1). The problem provides information about the patient's reason for seeking physical therapy services. This information helps the PT in making decisions regarding what information to seek during the history-taking and what tests and measures to include in the objective examination process. Following this initial record of "Problem," the subjective information is written.

## Structure

It should be evident that appropriate documentation of the subjective information will require some type of structure. Due to the amount and diversity of subjective information, if the data were recorded in a narrative form, it would be very difficult for the therapist to be able to analyze the data and compare the information to data gathered during the objective examination and during future re-examinations. Without an identifiable structure, other health care providers, auditors, and third party payers will have difficulty finding the information they are seeking. A narrative format would make it cumbersome for the PT to demonstrate the correlations between the subjective data, the objective data, the assessment, and the plan of care. To avoid these problems, the subjective information should be organized by grouping similar information together. It is helpful to utilize subheadings to help categorize the information and allow for quicker and easier identification of information. Although there is no universal standard for subheadings or for the organization of the subheadings, the therapist should present the information in a logical fashion that will help paint a clear clinical picture of the patient as well as the issues that will impact the patient's episode of care. The categories identified for history information presented in *The Guide to Physical Therapist Practice* are examples of subheadings that can be utilized. Refer to Table 6-2 for examples.

## Tips

When recording subjective information, the therapist should indicate the source of the data—whether it is the medical record, the patient, or a family member/caregiver. Often individuals will differentiate information gleaned from the medical record from that gathered from the patient or family member by using the subheading "medical record" or "medical chart." When practicing in an inpatient facility, it is tempting to review the medical record for information but not include the information in the PT documentation. Therapists may try to rationalize this omission by stating that the information is already available in the chart so there is no need to rewrite it in the physical therapy note. However, this approach is not advisable. Although it is true that physical therapy care is provided in concert with other disciplines and medical interventions and therefore must demonstrate the interrelationship between physical therapy services and other services, it is equally true that physical

---

**Example 1**

*ANYTOWN COMMUNITY HOSPITAL*
*SUBACUTE REHABILITATION*

*Physical Therapy Evaluation*

**Patient**:  D.W.
**Date**:     05/26/07
**Referral**: Physical therapy to evaluate and treat as advised
**Referring**
**Physician**: Dr. Sue Morton

Pr: Brainstem CVA 05/21/06; Type 2 diabetes; (R) carotid endarterectomy 07/04, and three previous TIA's.

S: <u>General Demographics</u>: 68 y/o Caucasian female, college education
<u>Current Condition</u>: Pt. reports that on 05/21/07 she awoke to find she could not get herself out of bed.  She had been experiencing feelings of fatigue and weakness the evening before and had gone to bed early.  Pt.'s husband called emergency services and she was transported to the hospital where the diagnosis of brainstem CVA was made.
<u>Patient Complaint</u>: Pt. c/o weakness on the (R) side of her body and "clumsiness" with her (L) arm.  States she is unable to lift anything on her own at this point.  Pt. admits to being very frustrated and just "wants to give up."
<u>Living Environment/Social Support</u>: Pt. reports she previously lived at home with her husband in a one-story ranch style home with 1 step to enter. The pt. and her husband have three children. One son lives in the area and can be available to assist on occasion. The other two children do not live in the area. Her husband owns his own business as an electrician and will be able to cut back his work hours to help her if needed.
<u>Prior level of function/activities</u>: Pt. states she has always been a "housewife" and is sure her husband would be unable to "run the home". Pt's social activities include going out to eat with friends approximately once a week and attending church twice a week. Pt. also reports she occasionally keeps her neighbor's children in the evenings. The children are 5 and 8 years old.
<u>Patient's goals</u>: She states she and her husband are hoping that she can eventually return home. She would like to return to as many of her previous activities as possible but voices she understands she may need to use a cane, walker or wheelchair to get around. Pt. is most concerned about being able to take care of her home including doing dishes, laundry, and general housecleaning tasks.

---

therapy services are separate from other interventions and services. Because of this, it is imperative that the physical therapy process should have clear documentation. The clinical problem-solving process used by the PT needs to be clearly identifiable in order to demonstrate medical necessity and the need for skilled care as is directly related to physical therapy. The physical therapy examination and evaluation documentation should refer to other disciplines and data as appropriate but should also be a stand-alone document. Regardless of the forms or formats that are utilized in a particular facility, the therapist is responsible for ensuring that the documentation contains all pertinent information to support the clinical decisions when creating the physical therapy diagnosis, prognosis, and plan of care.[5-6]

When writing the subjective information, the following verbs will commonly be used: states, reports, denies, and describes. As in, "The patient reports having pain in his left shoulder." Or, "The patient denies any previous surgeries." When possible, the therapist should use quotes to demonstrate the patient's cogni-

tive or emotional status or attitude toward therapy. For example, a 48-year-old female patient who is receiving physical therapy due to an exacerbation of multiple sclerosis with significant functional decline is showing signs of depression. The therapist documents the patient's quote, "I am just getting tired of all of this. I don't think I have it in me to take much more." Documentation of this quote will provide evidence for conclusions the therapist may draw about the patient's affective response to her disease that will be recorded in the assessment portion of the note and will facilitate the patient receiving appropriate medical treatment.

When documenting in a physical therapy report, the information must be presented in a way that is easy to read and understand; however, strict grammatical guidelines do not always have to be observed. Often a series of data pieces will be presented in sentence structure that would be considered a sentence fragment. As long as the sentences are complete enough to detail the information that needs to be documented and the sentences are located within a subheading that helps to provide the context to the information, "complete" sentences are not necessary. For example, there is no need to repeat the phrase, "The pt. reports...."

# How to Use Subjective Information

As discussed above, the first use of subjective information is to further inform the examination process and guide the therapist in determining other subjective data to gather and specific tests and measures to perform. For example, while interviewing a 56-year-old male, he reports pain in his low back. The therapist will then alter the history-taking to include asking detailed questions about the patient's back pain (frequency, duration, description, exact location, aggravating factors, etc.). The therapist will also make a mental note of several tests and measures to include (range of motion measurements, palpation of structures, observation of functional activities, etc.) within the objective portion of the examination.

The subjective information will also be used as a benchmark for future assessment. As interventions are provided, the PT or physical therapist assistant (PTA) will review the subjective data from the evaluation to determine the patient's progress.

## The Physical Therapist Assistant and the S: Section

The PTA will use the subjective portion of the initial evaluation to get a better picture of what to expect when interacting with the patient. The PTA should be familiar with the subjective information in the event that the patient reveals new data that should be reported to the PT. For example, a PTA is working with a 78-year-old female who fell and fractured her pelvis. The initial evaluation indicated that the patient was planning on returning home to her apartment alone upon discharge. During a follow-up session, the patient shared that her plans had changed and she would be traveling out of state to live close to her children. The PTA will document this information and inform the PT of the patient's change of plans so the PT can determine if adjustments to the plan of care are necessary. The PTA also uses the subjective information from the initial evaluation to determine what questions to be prepared to ask the patient during interim visits. For example, a patient is receiving outpatient therapy services for a shoulder injury. During the initial evaluation, the patient reports he is unable to reach up into the cabinets to get a glass. The PTA will note this and remember to ask the patient about his ability to perform this functional activity during subsequent therapy sessions.

# Summary

The subjective, or "S:" section of the SOAP note is the documentation of information gleaned during the history-taking portion of the examination. This information is useful in informing the remainder of the examination process as well as providing pertinent data upon which the therapist will draw conclusions about the diagnosis, prognosis, and plan of care. Documenting subjective information in a logical structure will help inform and show the clinical decision-making process by providing a framework for review and comparison of future data collected. Now that a comprehensive history-taking has occurred and appropriate subjective information has been gathered and documented, we can turn our attention to the systems review and tests and measures portion of the examination and discuss documentation of the objective data.

---

*Questions a PTA will ask when reviewing the subjective portion of a SOAP note:*

- *"What do I need to know to be able to effectively work with this patient?"* The PTA will be looking for the medical diagnosis, any precautions/contraindications, body structure or body function impairments, functional or activity limitations, or disabilities/participation restrictions. This information (along with the remainder of the evaluative note) will provide the PTA with a picture of what to expect when working with the patient.

- *"What other diagnosis does this patient have that might impact performance in physical therapy?"* A patient recovering from a hip fracture that underwent an ORIF and must follow restricted weight bearing precautions may also have a diagnosis of Alzheimer's disease. Due to cognitive dysfunction, this patient will have difficulty maintaining the correct weight bearing.

- *"What questions do I need to be prepared to ask the patient?"* If the evaluative note indicates the patient reported being in pain the PTA will want to ask the patient about his or her pain level.

- *"What type of responses might cause me to decide not to initiate treatment, to stop treatment once it has started, or to consult with the physical therapist?"* If the patient indicates a new source or type of pain, the PTA will be prepared to respond appropriately.

# Review Questions

1. Describe the types of information that should be documented in the subjective portion of a SOAP note.

2. Identify appropriate sources for obtaining subjective information. Compare and contrast the validity of each source.

3. Discuss the relationship between the subjective examination and the objective examination.

4. Discuss the relationship between the subjective examination and the evaluation process.

5. Create a diagram that demonstrates the relationship between the subjective examination, the objective examination, diagnosis, prognosis, and plan of care.

6. What is the value of subjective information that is not used for diagnostic reasons?

7. How will the PTA use the subjective information found within the evaluative note? How can the PT structure the note to enhance the PT/PTA relationship?

8. Outline an appropriate structure for the documentation of subjective information.

# Application Exercises

1. Interview a PT. Ask him or her to reflect on a situation when the subjective information provided by the patient significantly impacted his or her clinical decisions.

2. Interview a PTA. Ask him or her to discuss how he or she uses the subjective information from an evaluative note.

3. For the following information, indicate an appropriate subheading.
   a. pain complaints
   b. age
   c. number of steps into the home
   d. ability to ambulate prior to surgery
   e. work tasks
   f. reports of seeking care from a chiropractor
   g. hand dominance
   h. patient's mother died of a stroke
   i. patient is unmarried
   j. results of blood work

4. Indicate the preferred source (patient, patient's family member/caregiver, patient's medical chart) to obtain the following information and describe why that is the preferred source.
   a. number of steps leading into the home
   b. type of surgery that was performed
   c. description of pain
   d. patient's ability to get in/out of bed
   e. patient's prior health status
   f. current medications
   g. sleep patterns
   h. patient's adjustment to a permanent disability
   i. distance from the bed to the bathroom
   j. school-related expectations for a pediatric client

5. Write the following statements in a more clear and concise manner, as it would appear in the medical record. Also, indicate the subheading the information would fall under.

a. The patient said that her pain was three out of ten on a pain scale.

b. The patient said he is planning to return home after he is released from the hospital.

c. The patient's wife said that the patient has not been able to get up out of bed by himself for the past two weeks.

d. The patient said he has not been able to complete his work tasks because he gets tired and has to sit down about every five minutes.

e. The patient's husband tells the therapist that to get from the car to the house the patient will have to walk about 25 feet over grass and then will need to go up four steps and that the steps do not have a railing.

6. Organize the following information so that it is clear, concise and suitable for entry into the medical record.

a. Mr. Jones tells you that he hurt his hand in a work accident. Since the accident, he says his fingers have started to swell very badly. He says that he has pain at a level of 7 out of a 10 point scale. He says he has not been able to make a fist and has had difficulty with getting dressed and eating due to the swelling and pain in his hand.

b. Mrs. Pearson's son has brought her to see a therapist in an outpatient clinic. The patient's son says the patient has had difficulty sleeping at night due to hip pain. He also says he has had to help his mother "limp around the house," and says that she is having a lot of pain and is fearful of falling. The patient says that because of the pain she feels like her hip is going to "give out" when she stands.

c. A patient with a diagnosis of bicipital tendonitis has been referred to you by her physician. The patient says her pain is a 3 on a 10 point scale at the time of the examination. The patient says that she is having trouble reaching into overhead cabinets and shelves. The patient indicates that she is a cashier at a grocery store and says she has been off work due to the pain. She says that when she works the pain gets unbearable and says it is a 12 on a 10 point scale.

d. A 17-year-old patient is in a coma after a motor vehicle accident. The patient's mother states that the patient is very active and is involved in basketball and baseball. The mother says the patient was attending college at the local university and has been living in the dorm. The mother states the patient has been responding to her by squeezing her hand but that the patient has not said anything to her.

e. A 98-year-old patient is being seen in his apartment through home health services. The patient says he is occasionally a "little wobbly" but that he doesn't think he needs "all this attention." The patient says he has not fallen. He says that he is very careful and he takes his time getting around his house. He states, "I don't need to be in any hurry, I don't have nowhere to go. I did all my hurrying when I was a young man." The patient says he would rather not participate in physical therapy.

7. Review the subjective portion of a SOAP note as found in Example 2. Critique the note and answer the following questions. Is any critical information missing? Does the documentation address impairments, functional limitations, and disabilities? What questions would the therapist need to ask to gain the additional information needed? Where would the therapist get this information (what source—this may include people)?

8. Rewrite the subjective portion of the SOAP note as found in Example 2, organizing the information so that it is clear, concise, and suitable for entry into the medical record.

9. While performing an examination of a patient, the following information is obtained. Organize and write the information so that it is clear, concise, and suitable for entry into the medical record.

The patient is in a skilled nursing facility. The patient had a total hip replacement surgery 4 days ago. The medical record indicates the patient is 67 years old and has a past medical history that includes degenerative joint disease of both of her shoulders as well as has had hypertension that she has been treated for over the past 8 years. The patient also had two previous transischemic attacks within the last 2 years. The patient was admitted for a total hip replacement due to radiologic findings of severe degeneration of her left hip as well as reports from the patient that she was having difficulty with getting around in her home. The patient is on the following medications: Percocet, Plavix, Toprol XL, and Senokot S. The patient reports that she is having general soreness from lying around so much and states

## Example 2

*Outpatient Physical Therapy Initial Evaluation*

**Patient's Name**: D.T.
**Evaluation Date**:        July 12, 2006
**Referring Diagnosis**: S/P Left Patellectomy

**Subjective**: This is a 38 y/o male with a long history of (L) knee problems.  Patient initially fell injuring his knee on 9/04/04.  He subsequently underwent arthroscopy in October 2004 followed with approximately three weeks of physical therapy.  Patient underwent patellectomy in Jan 2005, followed by extensive therapy from March to July 2005.  At that time, the patient was discharged to a home exercise program, which he states he has been performing consistently since that time. The patient was seen by Dr. Sundstrom approximately 6/21/06. He presented to this clinic with orders for aggressive rehab with no restrictions.  Patient was scheduled in and was not seen until this date secondary to several falls and difficulty with the knee.  This has been a primary problem for this patient and indeed he did stop by the department one day after sustaining one of these falls to cancel his initial appointment. The patient's chief complaint is that of weakness and pain in the (L) knee.

she is having moderate pain in her hip, which she rates as a 4 on a 10 point scale. The patient says that she is a retired school teacher and that she spends her time caring for her home and her garden. She says that she lives in a house with her husband. She reports that her husband is in good health and can help around the house some but that he is "no homemaker and might even burn supper given the chance." She says that she has three grown children and four grandchildren. The patient indicates that only one of her children lives in the area. Her daughter that lives in the area works full-time and will not be able to provide any assistance. The patient describes her home as a ranch style home with one step to enter. The patient indicates that she is active in her church and participates with a book club that meets every Thursday morning at a local coffee shop. The patient reports that she and her husband enjoy traveling and that they have plans to travel to Rome this summer. The patient says she has never smoked and that she drinks alcohol socially.

# References

1. American Physical Therapy Association. *The Guide to Physical Therapist Practice.* Alexandria, VA: APTA; 2001.
2. Merriam-Webster's Online Dictionary. www.m-w.com/dictionary/subjective. Accessed on 11/13/06.
3. Edwards I, Jones M, Carr J, Braunack-Mayer A, Jensen G, Clinical Reasoning Strategies in Physical Therapy. *Phys Ther.* 2004;84(4):312-330.
4. World Health Organization. *International Classification of Functioning, Disability and Health.* Geneva. 2001
5. Stewart DL, Abeln, SH. *Documenting Functional Outcomes in Physical Therapy.* St. Louis, MO: Mosby; 1993.
6. Lewis K. Do The Write Thing: Document Everything. *PT - Magazine of Physical Therapy.* 2002;10(7):30-34.

## Chapter 7

# Recording Objective Information

*Rebecca McKnight, PT, MS*

## Chapter Objectives

Upon completion of this chapter, the reader will be able to:

1. Identify types of data that should be recorded in the objective portion of a SOAP note.
2. Discuss the purpose of the systems review.
3. Discuss the clinical decision-making process used to determine which tests and measures to perform.
4. Discuss how objective data is used to inform the clinical decision-making process.
5. Differentiate between measurements of impairments in body structure and function, a functional or activity limitation, or a disability/participation restriction.
6. Explain the rationale for including objective data with "normal findings" within the documentation that indicates no impairment or functional deficit exists.
7. Arrange data collected during the objective portion of an examination into a logically sequenced, objective note.
8. Discuss how the physical therapist assistant will use the objective information found in an initial evaluative note.

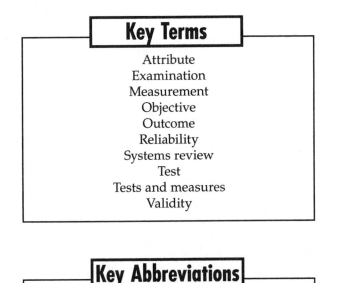

### Key Terms
Attribute
Examination
Measurement
Objective
Outcome
Reliability
Systems review
Test
Tests and measures
Validity

### Key Abbreviations
O:

| | Table 7-1 |
|---|---|
| Correlation Between Objective Portion of a SOAP Note and APTA's Patient/Client Management Model | |
| **Patient/Client Management Model** | *SOAP Evaluative Note* |
| **Examination** | |
| • History | Problem (Pr:) Subjective (S:) |
| • Systems Review • Tests and Measurements | Objective (O:) |
| **Evaluation Diagnosis Prognosis** | Assessment (A:) |
| **Intervention** | Plan (P:) |

# Introduction

Chapter 6 discussed the portion of the physical therapist's examination known as history-taking and outlined the method for documenting the subjective portion of the SOAP note. An overview of the variety of types of data that should be considered and how these data inform the remainder of the physical therapy process was examined. For instance, the information received during the subjective portion of the exam will inform the remainder of the examination process. After completion of the history-taking, the physical therapist (PT) will begin collecting data through two steps: 1) reviewing body systems, and 2) performing tests and measures. In this chapter, both of these examination components will be reviewed and techniques for appropriate documentation of the results will be given.

# What Is Objective Information?

Objective information includes data gathered during the "'hands-on' component of the examination"[1(p34)] (Table 7-1). These pieces of data are gathered through the physical therapist's direct observation. Objective data are obtained through various methods and techniques such as range of motion (ROM) measurements, gross muscle testing, sensation testing, girth measurements, and functional tests. When possible, these methods are based on clearly defined procedures and are therefore reproducible. Using reproducible methods helps to ensure validity and reliability of the data obtained. Objective data must have some measure of reliability and be useful in supporting the clinical decision-making process.

During the examination process, a therapist should collect data from a general systems review as well as from specific tests and measures. Data gathered during these two components of the examination will be used in conjunction with the data gathered during the subjective portion of the examination to determine the physical therapy diagnosis, prognosis, and intervention. Further, the objective data will also be used as a reference to evaluate outcomes and note the patient's progress throughout the episode of care.

The other category of information that is documented within the objective portion of a SOAP note is any intervention that is provided. In most cases, the patient will receive some intervention during the initial therapy session. These interventions should be documented within the evaluative note. Methods and tips for documenting interventions will be expanded upon in Chapter 9 (Figure 7-1).

# Systems Review

*The Guide to Physical Therapist Practice* defines a systems review as a "brief or limited examination of: (1) the anatomical and physiological status of the cardiovascular/pulmonary, integumentary, musculoskeletal, and neuromuscular systems, and (2) the communication ability, affect, cognition, language, and learning style of the patient."[1(p34)] The purpose of the systems review is to gain an overall picture of the patient and his or her health. It provides the opportunity to screen all of the systems that will impact the patient's participation in physical therapy and will help the therapist in determining more specific tests and measures to utilize. Data gleaned from the systems review may also point to the need for referral to other health care providers and is therefore an essential part of the examination process for an autonomous practitioner. The following are examples of the types of data that are gathered during a systems review.

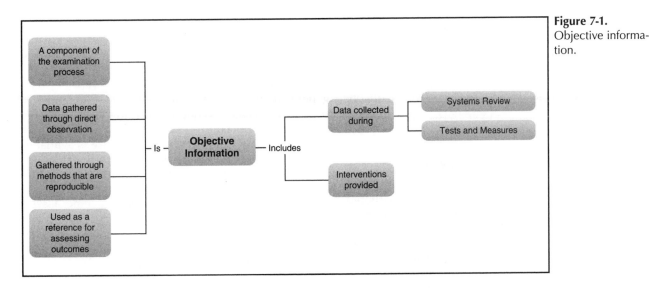

**Figure 7-1.**
Objective information.

## Cardiovascular/Pulmonary System

- Heart rate (recorded as beats per minutes).
- Respiratory rate (recorded as breaths per minute).
- Blood pressure (must include patient position and location where BP is taken, eg, (R) UE).
- Edema in the extremities.

## Integumentary System

- Skin integrity (noting any areas of loss of skin integrity such as scrapes, cuts, or open wounds).
- Skin color (specifically noting color abnormalities or changes such as redness around bony landmarks that might indicate development of a pressure sore).
- Presence of scar formation (this should include surgical scars and should indicate the location and appearance of each scar).

## Musculoskeletal System

- Gross symmetry (noting things such as leg length discrepancies and postural deficits such as a forward head or rounded shoulders).
- Gross ROM (noting patient's ability to move extremities through available range).
- Gross strength (as noted through a gross strength screening looking at overall muscle group function).
- Height
- Weight

## Neuromuscular System

- Gross coordination of movements (can be noted primarily through observation of the patient during functional tasks).
- Balance (noting general balance function during sitting and standing).
- Locomotion (ability to walk or use a wheelchair, taking note of assistive devices used, distance, surfaces, and level of assist provided by the therapist).
- Transfers (movement from one surface to another, ie, sit to stand; noting assistive or adaptive equipment and level of assist provided by the therapist).
- Transitions (movement in bed from one position to another, ie, rolling over in bed; noting assistive or adaptive equipment and level of assist provided by the therapist).

## Other

- Communication ability (noting any signs of aphasia or other communication deficits such as hearing or speech impairments).
- Affect (noting observable signs of affect such as crying, laughing, apprehensive movements, etc.)
- Cognition (noting any cognitive problems such as loss of orientation to self, place, or time).
- Language (noting if the patient has a primary language other than English and the ability to speak/comprehend English if it is not the primary language).

- Learning style (noting the patient's preference for receiving information, i.e. demonstration, verbal instruction, or written instruction.
- Ability to make needs known
- Level of consciousness (ie, alert, drowsy, unconscious, etc.)[1](p34-35)

# Tests and Measures

Objective information also includes data gathered utilizing specific tests and measures. These tests and measures are "used to rule in or out causes of impairment and functional limitations; to establish a diagnosis, prognosis and plan of care; and to select interventions."[1](p35) These measurements are also used as baseline data upon which outcome data is compared to determine the patient's response to interventions. Tests and measures are selected based upon the information collected from the history-taking as well as from the systems review. A large variety of tests and measures are available for use by the PT. It is not within the scope of this text to discuss in detail issues related to tests and measures and appropriate selection per case. However, basic concepts that should be kept in mind when selecting specific tests or measurements will be outlined here and expanded upon in Chapter 10.

A *test* is a specified procedure used to gather identifiable data (the measurement) and a *measurement* is the label (or categorization) given to a specific attribute being observed.[2] Rothstein and Echternach state in *Primer on Measurement: An Introductory Guide to Measurement Issues*, "No measurement should be obtained unless there is an identified attribute, characteristic, property, dimension, or variable to be categorized or quantified. In other words, you should not attempt to measure something unless you know what that something is."[2](p7) Appropriate selection of the specific test or measure to perform must first begin by identifying the attribute to be quantified or measured. Once the attribute has been determined, the therapist can determine what available tests and measurement tools to use. The attribute being measured may be at the impairment level, the functional level, or at the disability/participation restriction level. For example, an individual's lower extremity strength may be measured at the body structure/function level by utilizing a handheld dynamometer[3](p2-3) or at the activity limitations level by having the patient perform multiple sit to stand transfers.[4]

As part of the selection process, the therapist should consider the validity and reliability of the test and measurement tool. When a therapist utilizes valid and reliable tools, the credibility of the interpretation and the ability to determine the prognosis, diagnosis, and plan of care are improved. An exhaustive list of tests and measures is beyond the scope of this text-book. However, examples have been provided based upon categories of tests and measures as listed in *The Guide for Physical Therapist Practice*. For a more comprehensive listing of the types of tests and measures, the tools/instruments that can be utilized, types of data generated, validity, and reliability of the methods, refer to *The Guide*.[1] When performing tests and measures, it is important to use standardized procedures when available. If no standard procedure is available, or if the case demands an alteration to the standard procedure, it is imperative to document the procedure being used in clear detail so the procedure can be repeated in the future for reliable outcome assessment.

---

*Definitions related to tests and measures:*

*Attribute*: a variable; a characteristic or quality that is measured.

*Examination*: a test or a group of tests used for the purpose of obtaining measurements or data.

*Measurement*: the numeral assigned to an object, event, or person or the class (category) to which an object, event, or person is assigned according to rules.

*Test*: a procedure or set of procedures that is used to obtain measurements (data); the procedures may require the use of instruments.

*Practicality of a test*: the usefulness of a test based on issues relating to personnel, time, equipment, cost of administration, and impact on the person taking the test.

*Reliability*: the consistency or repeatability of measurements; the degree to which measurements are error-free and the degree to which repeated measurements will agree.

*Validity*: the degree to which a useful (meaningful) interpretation can be inferred from a measurement.[2]

---

## Aerobic Capacity/Endurance

- Response to activity: heart rate, respiratory rate, blood pressure, oxygen saturation (indicate when these measurements are taken—before or after activity)
- Respiratory rate (include rate, rhythm, depth, and regularity of pattern).
- Activities of daily living (ADL) scales

- Step tests
- Electrocardiography
- Auscultation
- Perceived exertion scales

## Anthropometric Characteristics

- Body composition (body mass index, skin-fold thickness measurement)
- Weight
- Length (determining length discrepancies)
- Girth for edema measurement or to examine muscle mass
- Volumetric displacement to monitor edema

## Arousal, Attention, and Cognition

- Arousal and attention
- Cognition (ability to process commands)
- Communication
- Consciousness (level of agitation, coma scales)
- Orientation (to person, place, time and situation)

## Assistive and Adaptive Devices

- Specify device being used during specific functional tasks
- Describe patient's (patient's family/caregiver's) ability to care for device
- Describe patient's ability to don/doff device as appropriate
- Describe skin condition related to use of the device
- Describe safety risks associated with use of the device

## Circulation

- Heart rate (includes location, quality and rate per minute).
- Blood pressure (include location, eg, right vs. left and indicate systolic over diastolic)
- Claudication scales
- Palpation

## Cranial and Peripheral Nerve Integrity

- Electrophysiological integrity
- Dynamometry
- Tension tests
- Provocation tests

- Discrimination test (tactile tests including cold and heat, pain, pressure)

## Environmental, Home, and Work (Job/School/Play) Barriers

- Questionnaires
- Photographic assessment
- Observations
- Description of barriers, environment

## Ergonomics and Body Mechanics

- Manipulative ability tests
- Impairment rating scales
- Functional capacity tests
- Hazard identification checklists
- Job severity indexes
- Job simulations
- Vibration assessments

## Gait, Locomotion, and Balance

- Describe activity
- Indicate any assistive, adaptive, orthotic, protective, supportive, or prosthetic devices used
- Indicate type of surface the patient is traversing
- Indicate distance traveled or amount of time activity is tolerated
- List amount and type of physical assistance provided

  Examples include:
  - supervision: no physical contact needed
  - contact guard assist (CGA): a hand on the patient but no physical assist provided
  - minimal assist [min (a), min @, or min (A)]: the therapist provides 25% assistance to the patient
  - moderate assist [mod (a), mod @, or mod (A)]: the therapist provides 50% assistance to the patient
  - maximal assist [max (a), max @, or max (A)]: the therapist provides 75% assistance to the patient
  - dependent (D): the therapist provides 100% of the effort and the patient does not physically participate
- Number of people needed to provide assistance

- When using min, mod, and max assist to describe the amount of assistance provided to the patient, also include the number of individuals providing the assist, eg, min (A) x 2 indicates that two individuals provided minimal assist
- List amount and type of cues given
  - verbal cues: Verbal instructions required only
- Describe gait pattern used if appropriate
  - Step to
  - Step through or swing through
- Describe gait deviations if appropriate, ie, foot slap at initial contact, toe drag during swing phase
- When documenting gait, include weight bearing status
  - Full weight bearing (FWB): 100% weight bearing.
  - Partial weight bearing (PWB): the patient is able to apply some weight to the involved extremity. Partial weight bearing usually indicates 50% unless otherwise indicated, eg, PWB 25% would indicate that the patient was able to bear 25% of his or her body weight through the involved extremity.
  - Toe touch weight bearing (TTWB): the patient is allowed to place his or her toes on the floor during gait for balance, but should not bear weight through the extremity.
  - Weight bearing as tolerated (WBAT): the patient is allowed to place as much weight on the extremity as his or her pain level will allow.
- ADL scales
- Dizziness inventory
- Fall scales
- Footprint analysis
- Videographic assessment
- Dynamic posturography

## Integumentary Integrity

- Location of wound/skin condition
- Size of wound
- Depth of wound
- Location and depth of any tunneling/undermining
- Description of tissue (eg, color, healthy, unhealthy, granulating, necrotic, etc.)

- Description of surrounding area (eg, dry, moist, shiny, macerated, color, temperature, texture, etc.)
- Description of drainage (eg, clear, bloody, thick, thin, serous, etc.)
- Description of odor
- Record activities, positioning, and postures that aggravate or relieve pain or altered sensation, or that produce associated skin trauma
- Photographic assessment
- Pressure-sensing maps

## Joint Integrity and Mobility

- Describe abnormal joint movements/end feels
- Apprehension tests
- Valgus/varus stress test

## Motor Function (Motor Control and Motor Learning)

- Coordination screens
- Motor proficiency tests
- Electroneuromyography
- Dexterity tests
- Developmental scales
- Movement assessment batteries

## Muscle Performance (Including Strength, Power, and Endurance)

- Dynamometry
- Manual muscle tests
- Timed activity tests
- ADL scales
- Palpation

## Neuromotor Development and Sensory Integration

- Developmental inventories and questionnaires
- Infant and toddler motor assessments
- Reflex tests
- Behavioral assessment scales
- Visual perceptual skills tests

## Orthotic, Protective, and Supportive Devices

- Observation of component alignment and fit
- Pressure-sensing maps
- ADL scales
- Pain scales
- Fall scales

## Pain

- Pain questionnaires, scales, and diagrams
- Structural provocation tests

## Posture

- Observation of alignment of trunk
- Observation of alignment of extremities in relation to the trunk
- Grid measurement
- Forward-bending test
- Photographic assessment

## Prosthetic Requirements

- Observation of component alignment and fit
- Observation of ability to don/doff prosthesis
- ADL scale
- Functional performance inventory
- Goniometry
- Muscle tests

## Range of Motion (Including Muscle Length)

- Observation of functional ROM
- Goniometry
- Inclinometry
- Muscle length test

## Reflex Integrity

- Myotatic reflex scale
- Electroneuromyography
- Observation of postural reflexes
- Observation of primitive reflexes

## Self-Care and Home Management

- Record measurements of physical environments

- Record any safety concerns or barriers in home
- Physical performance tests
- ADL scales

## Sensory Integrity

- Stereognosis tests
- Vibration tests
- Electroneuromyography

## Ventilation and Respiration/Gas Exchange

- Gas analyses
- Pulmonary function tests
- Ventilatory muscle force tests
- Breath and voice sounds
- Dyspnea

## Work (Job/School/Play), Community, and Leisure Integration or Reintegration

- Observation of ability to resume work activities
- Physical capacity tests
- Barrier identification
- Observation of safety with activities in work, community, and leisure activity environments[1(p48-95)]

# Importance of Documenting Objective Information

Objective data provides the primary foundation upon which the diagnosis and prognosis will be based. This data, along with data from the historytaking, will be used to determine the plan of care. Since objective data is gathered through reproducible procedures, the information is verifiable and therefore useful for validating the need for physical therapy services. Objective data is the information to which future measurements can be compared to demonstrate the patient's progress throughout the episode of care.

Objective data is used to form a detailed picture of the patient and the problem and is used to guide the physical therapy decision-making process. It is important to remember that the primary goal of physical therapy should be to impact the individual at the activity/functional limitation or participation/

disability level. Therefore, documentation of objective data should indicate how function has been affected. This does not mean that information at the impairment level is not valuable; however, only gathering impairment-related data greatly limits the therapist's view of the patient's condition. It is not advisable to draw direct conclusions about the patient's ability to function or participate within his or her normal environment utilizing only information about impairments in the patient's body functions and body structures. The therapist will have the opportunity to indicate relationships between impairments, functional/activity limitations, and disabilities/participation restrictions within the assessment portion of the document.

Documentation of function is imperative within current practice guidelines. Reimbursement is typically tied to improvement in function, thus documentation of limitations in a patient's functional abilities helps to justify the need for physical therapy services. Focus on function also helps with patient motivation since functional activities are more meaningful to patients. For example, a patient is not as interested in how many degrees of motion she has available in her shoulder joint except as it correlates with her ability to comb her hair.

## Limitations of Objective Data

The degree to which objective data are limited is related in part to the availability of reliable and valid tools for the measurement of the specific attribute. A highly reliable measurement may be obtained, but it may provide limited insight into the patient's functional mobility. For example, goniometric measurement of the knee can provide reliable data related to the amount of ROM available at the knee joint,[5(p39-48)] but this information does not give direct information related to the functional ambulatory status of the patient. In recent years, there has been a focus on the development of a variety of tests and measures for the assessment of functional mobility to provide more direct measures of patients' functional abilities.

It should be remembered that one measurement of a single attribute will not provide adequate data to support the determination of a diagnosis, prognosis, or appropriate plan of care. Typically, multiple pieces of data are required to provide the information necessary for clinical decision-making. Much like one piece of a puzzle rarely provides enough detail to determine the whole picture, one piece of data will not provide an adequate view of the patient or the problem to result in informed clinical decisions. The physical therapy diagnosis, prognosis, and plan of care are determined by an accumulation of pieces of information. The aggregate data require the clinical reasoning of a PT to interpret its significance. This activity is known as the evaluation and will be discussed in further detail in Chapter 8.

# How to Document Objective Information

## Structure

There is no strict standard structure for documentation of objective data. However, the information should be presented in a logical sequence in order to assist the therapist in the clinical decision-making process and to allow reviewers of the documentation to be able to determine the PT's clinical reasoning process.

To allow for easy identification of data, it is necessary to organize the information with the use of subheadings. The choice of subheadings can either be determined by the clinical facility or it can be left up to the discretion of the PT. Often, subheadings will vary depending upon the type of setting (acute hospital vs. home health) or the type of condition (neuromuscular vs. cardiopulmonary/vascular). For example, an acute care setting will frequently necessitate a subheading for "bed-mobility" within documentation, while an outpatient setting may rarely require the utilization of that subheading. Common subheadings used include: general observation, vital signs, strength, range of motion, and functional mobility. Alternately, the categories listed in *The Guide to Physical Therapist Practice* can also function as appropriate subheadings.

When documenting interventions that have been provided, it is important to clearly distinguish the intervention data from the tests and measurement data. This can be accomplished by separating tests and measurement data from the interventions data and by clearly labeling the interventions as such. Documentation of interventions will be discussed in further detail in Chapter 9.

Often, information in the objective section is best communicated in a list, column, or table format. These formats are used to make the information easier to read and locate. Goniometric measurements, manual muscle testing, girth, and volumetric measurements are types of information that are frequently documented in this format.

## Tips

The precise method used to document individual tests and measurements varies. It is important for the physical therapist to be familiar with the standard documentation of the measurement for the test being used. For example, the standard method to document a strength measurement when using Manual Muscle Testing is to document the scale being used.

*Instead of documenting*: (R) elbow bicep strength: 3
*Use*: Strength: (R) biceps: 3/5

*Subheadings for objective data:*

- Aerobic capacity
- Anthropometric characteristics
- Arousal, attention, and cognition
- Circulation
- Cranial and peripheral nerve integrity
- Environmental, home, and work barriers
- Ergonomics and body mechanics
- Gait
- Locomotion
- Balance
- Integumentary integrity
- Joint integrity or mobility
- Motor function
- Muscle performance
- Neuromotor development and sensory integration
- Orthotic, protective, and supportive devices
- Pain
- Posture
- Prosthetic devices
- Range of motion
- Reflexes
- Self-care and home management skills
- Sensation
- Ventilation/respiration
- Work, community, or leisure status and integration or re-integration (including IADLs)[1]

Or when documenting goniometric measurements, the data should be given in a range.[5(p29-32)]

*Instead of documenting*: (R) elbow flexion PROM 45°
*Use*:  PROM: (R) elbow flexion 0 - 45°

When documenting results of tests and measures, it is important that all pertinent information be included to allow for reproduction of the test. Standard testing procedures will be assumed, and therefore if any alterations to the procedure are used these should be clearly detailed. Identifying the specific attribute being measured is equally important. For example, when documenting strength measures, the therapist should include the muscle or muscles being tested (individual or muscle group) and which extremity is being tested, as well as right or left side. The measurements should be arranged in a logical order and grouped anatomically, as in Example 1.

All data should be recorded in relationship to what the patient did, not what the therapist did. For example, when documenting gait the note would read:

Gait: Pt. ambulated 100' with a straight cane on level surfaces requiring mod (A) x 1

*Rather than*:
Gait: The PT walked the patient 100' providing mod (A)

As with subjective data, complete sentences are not a requirement, as in the above example. However, all pertinent information needs to be included.

Within the objective data, the therapist should document information that addresses the following three areas: 1) impairments, if any; 2) functional status, including abilities and limitations; and 3) participation in social roles and disabilities or participation restrictions. Documentation of both positive aspects (what the patient can do) as well as negative aspects (the patient's limitations) helps to provide a fully developed picture upon which clinical decision making can occur. Relationships between problems at the different levels should be delineated within the assessment portion of the note. Additionally, at least a brief statement should be written if there are no limitations in certain critical skills. For example, if the patient's muscle strength or muscle group strength is normal, the note would read:

Strength: (R) biceps 5/5
*or*
Strength: (L) LE 5/5

Never omit relevant normal findings. Also, you will need to use the phrase "within normal limits" (WNL) cautiously, and try not to get into a habit of documenting WNL rather than truly performing the test and documenting the findings. Normal findings can be documented within the systems review portion of the objective section when general screening has occurred, or they could be part of the more specific tests and measures portion of the examination. Documentation of normal findings within the tests and measures portion of the examination is appropriate when it is relevant to confirming, refuting, or reshaping the diagnosis.

Typical verbs to be used when documenting objective information include: *demonstrated, performed, appears* (as in visual appearance), and *is* (Example 2).

# How to Use Objective Information

During the subjective or history-taking portion of the examination, the therapist should begin to formulate a working hypothesis of the patient's problem

## Example 1

| | AROM | PROM | Strength |
|---|---|---|---|
| (R) hip abduction | 0 - 20° | 0 - 30° | 3-/5 |
| Adduction | 0° | 0 -10° | 2-/5 |
| Flexion | 0- 80° | 0 - 95° | 3-/5 |
| Extension | 0° | 0 - 5° | 2+/5 |
| (R) knee | 10 -100° | 5 - 120° | 3-/5 |
| (R) ankle DF | 0 - 5° | 0 - 20° | 3-/5 |
| PF | 0 - 45° | 0 - 45° | 4/5 |
| Inv | 0 - 20° | 0 - 30° | 3+/5 |
| Ev | 0 - 5° | 0 - 15° | 3+/5 |

(diagnosis) and prognosis. The therapist then selects tests and measures to perform that will help to rule in or rule out the clinical hypothesis. Analyzing these measurements is known as the *evaluation*. Documentation of the evaluation (the therapist's interpretation of the data) will occur within the assessment (A:) portion of the SOAP note. The objective data provide the evidence to support the therapist's clinical interpretations.

## The Physical Therapist Assistant and the O: section

Just as with the subjective information, the physical therapist assistant (PTA) will review the objective information to get a clear picture of what to expect when interacting with the patient. The PTA will use the objective data to determine the most appropriate approach to use with the patient. For example, if the objective data indicates the patient required significant verbal cues to complete a functional task, the PTA should be prepared to respond accordingly. The objective information will provide a foundation upon which future patient responses and progress during the intervention can be compared, so that the PTA can identify inappropriate or unexpected patient responses and can communicate these to the PT. Additionally, the PTA will review the objective information to determine what types of data need to be collected to demonstrate the patient's response to interventions provided. For example, if interventions to address edema are being used, the PTA will review the initial evaluation to determine whether girth measurements or volumetric measurements were used. The PTA will use the same test and measurement techniques used by the PT in order to obtain data that can be compared with the data from the initial evaluation.

## Summary

The objective section of the SOAP note is the documentation of information gleaned from direct observation by the PT during a systems review and tests and measures. The PT will evaluate the subjective and objective information to determine the physical therapy diagnosis, prognosis, and plan of care. The PT should attempt to utilize reliable and valid tests and measures whenever possible in order to add credibility to the decision making processes. Using tests that measure not only the impairments but that directly measure functional abilities and participation levels helps to gain a valuable view of the patient's condition and provides data upon which goals can be established and future performance can be compared. Information should be structured in a logical sequence to allow for ease of interpretation throughout the episode of care.

# Example 2

**Patient**: D.W.

**O:** <u>Systems Review</u>:
<u>Cardiovascular/Pulmonary System</u>:    BP: 128/70. HR: 74 bpm. RR: 20
<u>Integumentary System</u>:  Unimpaired.
<u>Musculoskeletal System</u>:  Gross ROM unimpaired. Gross strength impaired throughout trunk and (B) UE's & LE's (R) > (L).
<u>Neuromuscular System</u>:  Balance & motor control impaired throughout trunk and all four extremities. Functional mobility impaired for all tasks.
<u>Communication</u>:  Mild slurred speech. Pt. easily understood.
<u>Cognition</u>: Unimpaired.
<u>Other</u>: Urinary catheter noted

<u>Tests & Measures & Observation</u>:
<u>Observation</u>: Pt. grossly obese
<u>Sensory</u>:  Pt. demonstrates normal light & gross touch, pain/thermal and diminished proprioception/kinesthesia on (L) and mildly diminished light & gross touch, pain/thermal, and proprioception/kinesthesia on (R) throughout trunk and extremities.
<u>Tone</u>: The patient displayed mild hypotonia (R) UE & LE and normal tone (L) UE & LE.

| MMT: | (R) | (L) |
|---|---|---|
| Shoulder | | |
|     Flexors | 2/5 | 4/5 |
|     Extensors | 1/5 | 4/5 |
|     Abductors | 1/5 | 4/5 |
|     Adductors | 2/5 | 5/5 |
|     Medial Rotators | 2/5 | 5/5 |
|     Lateral Rotators | 1/5 | 4-/5 |
| Elbow | | |
|     Flexors | 2/5 | 5/5 |
|     Extensors | 0/5 | 4+/5 |
| Wrist | | |
|     Flexors | 1/5 | 4/5 |
|     Extensors | 0/5 | 4-/5 |
| Grip | 5# | 28# |
| Hip | | |
|     Flexors | 1/5 | 4-/5 |
|     Extensors | 3/5 | 4-/5 |
|     Abductors | 0/5 | 4-/5 |
|     Adductors | 3+/5 | 5/5 |
| Knee | | |
|     Flexors | 0/5 | 4/5 |
|     Extensors | 2+/5 | 5/5 |
| Ankle | | |
|     Dorsiflexors | 0/5 | 4+/5 |
|     Plantarflexors | 1/5 | 5/5 |

<u>Balance</u>:  Sitting static fair-, dynamic poor; Standing not assessed at this time.
<u>Coordination</u>:  Unable to assess (R) side due to weakness. (L) UE & LE demonstrates diminished coordination with all activities. Note apraxia and pass pointing during exercises.
<u>Bed mobility</u>:  Max (A) with rolling and scooting in bed in all directions.
<u>Transfers</u>:  Max (A) supine ↔ sit.  Unable to perform sit ↔ stand at this time. Bed ↔ mat or bed at this time is via Hoyer due to patient's large size, poor balance, and weakness.

*Questions a PTA will ask when reviewing the objective portion of a SOAP note:*

- *"What do I need to know to be able to effectively work with this patient?"* The PTA will be looking for any precautions/contraindications, body structure or body function impairments, functional or activity limitations or disabilities/participation restrictions. This will provide a picture of what the PTA can expect when working with the patient.
- *"What data do I need to collect to help demonstrate the patient's response to the treatment plan?"* Example: Monitoring blood pressure with a patient who is status post coronary artery bypass graft surgery
- *"What equipment do I need to provide the intervention?"* Example: Type of assistive device
- *"What type of responses might cause me to decide not to initiate treatment or to stop treatment once it has started or to consult with the physical therapist?"* Example: If the initial evaluation indicated a patient that recently had a stroke needed only minimal assistance with activities, the PT should be notified of the change in patient status if the PTA notes that the patient now requires maximal assistance.

# Review Questions

1. Describe the types of information that should be documented in the objective portion of a SOAP note.

2. Define reliability and validity. Describe how these issues impact the selection of tests and measures used during the examination process.

3. List the types of data obtained during the systems review process. How is this information used within the clinical decision-making process?

4. How are data from tests and measures used in clinical decision-making? How can limitations of objective data can be minimized and controlled?

5. What is the value of documenting data that is within normal limits?

6. How will the PTA use the objective information found within the evaluative note? How can the therapist structure the information to enhance the PT/PTA relationship?

7. When can tables or columns be used to document objective information? What are the benefits of structuring the information in this format?

8. Outline an appropriate structure for the documentation of objective information, including subheadings.

# Application Exercises

1. Review the list of categories for tests and measurements in *The Guide to Physical Therapist Practice*. Choose one category from tests and measures (eg, aerobic capacity and endurance) and identify one specific test/measure that can be used to collect data for that category. Identify the tools and procedures used for the test. Research the reliability and validity of that test. Indicate if the test measures an impairment or function, eg, disability, activity limitation, or participation restriction.

2. Write the following statements in a more clear and concise manner, as it would appear in the medical record.

   a. The patient walked 25 feet in the hallway of the hospital with the therapist lightly touching her back. She used a standard walker.

   b. The patient's strength was a 3 for the right quadriceps and a 4 for the left quadriceps.

   c. The patient demonstrated the following range of motion measurements: passive range of motion for the right shoulder flexion was 115° and for shoulder extension 10°.

   d. The patient propelled his wheelchair around the hospital, outside on the sidewalk, and up and down several ramps with the therapist providing verbal prompts for appropriate trunk positioning for going up and down the ramps.

   e. During the systems review, the measurements taken for the cardiovascular system were blood pressure at 135 systolic and 90 diastolic, heart rate at 98 beats per minute, the patient's oxygen saturation was 98%, and his respiratory rate was 12 breaths per minute.

3. Organize the following information so that it is clear, concise, and suitable for entry into the medical record.

   a. Right knee flexion 100°, right knee extension 5°, right hip abduction 20°, right hip flexion 100°, right ankle plantarflexion 20°, left elbow AROM 10°-100°, left shoulder flexion 100°, left shoulder abduction 100°, right hip internal rotation 20°, right ankle dorsiflexion 5°, left shoulder external rotation 60°, left shoulder internal rotation 45°, left hip abduction 25°, left hip extension 0°, right hip extension 5°, right elbow flexion 120°, right elbow extension 0°, right shoulder flexion 165°, left knee flexion 120°, left hip flexion 120°, left hip internal rotation 20°, left hip external rotation 40°, right hip external rotation 45°, left knee extension 0°, left plantarflexion 45°, left dorsiflexion 20°, right shoulder abduction 140°, right shoulder external rotation 80°, and right shoulder internal rotation 45°.

   b. The patient walked 10 feet twice with one person supplying 25% assistance. The patient used a standard walker and did not put any weight on the right leg. The therapist had to verbally remind the patient to place the walker forward 50% of the time. The patient walked in the hallway on level surfaces only.

   c. The patient walked with the therapist at his side (but not touching him) for 100 feet, twice. The patient's vital signs before walking were: blood pressure 125/85, respirations 15 per minute, and heart rate 77 beats per minute. The patient's vital signs after walking were: blood pressure 135/85, respirations 17 per minute, and heart rate 87 beats per minutes.

   d. Girth at the right knee joint line was 34 cm, 2 inches above was 38 cm, 4 inches above was 42 cm, and 4 inches below was 35.5 cm. Active flexion was 120°. The patient lacked 20° of active extension. Strength for the quad muscle was 3-/5 and for the hamstrings was 3/5. The patient walks independently with crutches, only putting his toe down for balance but not putting any weight through his lower extremity.

   e. Wound assessment revealed the following information. The skin around the wound is red, warm to the touch, shiny, and swollen. The wound is a 4 cm x 2.4 cm oval-shaped wound. It is 1.5 cm deep. The patient has diminished sensation to light touch when compared bilateral. She is unable to feel the 6.65 monofilament on the right. Girth at the right MTP joint is 22 cm and 18 cm on the left. The right dorsal pedis pulse is present but diminished compared to the (L) which is 2+.

4. Review the objective portion of a SOAP note as found in Example 3. Critique the note by answering the following questions:

   a. Is the information structured logically?

   b. Is the information presented in a way that allows for ease of finding pertinent information?

## Example 3

**Objective**:

<u>(L) Knee ROM</u>:

| | Active | Passive |
|---|---|---|
| Flexion: | 0° to 125° | 0° to 135° |
| Extension: | 0° to 0° | 0° to 0° |
| Hamstring Length: | in supine lacks 50° knee extension hip at 90° flexion | |
| Gastrocnemius Length: | in supine with knee fully extended 0 to 5° | |

<u>Strength</u>: (L) quadriceps 3-/5; (L) hamstrings 3/5; Patient has marked pain with resisted knee extension. Pain is most keenly felt over the mid portion of the patellar tendon.

<u>Gait</u>: Ambulates with one axillary crutch in the (R) hand and knee immobilizer in place. Gait noted after removal of the immobilizer, the patient keeps the affected knee in strict extension.

---

c. Does the objective information provide data that addresses body structures and body functions and impairments?

d. Does the objective information provide data about the patient's functional abilities or limitations?

e. Does the objective information provide data about the patient's activity participation or restrictions and disabilities?

f. What other data would be beneficial to gather?

5. While performing an examination of a patient who is recovering from a left total hip arthroplasty in a skilled nursing facility, the following information is obtained. Organize and write the information so that it is clear, concise, and suitable for entry into the medical record.

During the systems review, the following data were gathered: the blood pressure reading was 130/85, heart rate was 88 beats per minute and respiratory rate was 20 breaths per minute, there was a scar that appeared to be healing well on the left hip, surgical staples were present and intact and there was no drainage from the wound, during a gross muscle test the therapist noted a generalized decrease in strength in the uninvolved extremities and significant weakness was noted in the left leg. General range of motion was unrestricted except in the surgical limb, which was restricted to hip precautions per the orthopedic surgeon. The patient doesn't display any balance or coordination problems but does have difficulties with functional mobility. No problems were noted with the patient's ability to communicate or with the patient's cognitive abilities. The following measurements were taken during the tests and measures component of the examination. Manual muscle testing grades were four out of five to four plus out of five throughout the non-operative limbs. The left hip musculature was not tested due to the recent surgery and the patient's complaints of pain. The patient's left knee musculature measured at a three plus out of five and the ankle musculature measured five out of five. The therapist helped the patient walk in the hallway. The patient was able to walk 50 feet while the therapist provided about 25% assistance. The patient used a standard walker. The therapist provided verbal instructions for sequencing and encouragement to put as much weight as the patient felt comfortable with through the leg. The patient also occasionally placed the walker too far in front of her and the therapist had to remind the patient of the proper walker placement. When the therapist helped the patient up from the bed, the patient needed 25% assistance to scoot over in bed. The therapist primarily helped by moving the operative limb. When sitting on the side of the bed, the patient required more assistance and was able to perform about 50% of the activity. When moving from sitting on the edge of the bed to standing with the walker, the patient performed about 50% of the task.

# References

1. American Physical Therapy Association. *The Guide to Physical Therapist Practice.* Alexandria, VA: APTA; 2001.
2. Rothstein J, Echternach JL. *Primer on Measurement: An Introductory Guide to Measurement Issues.* Alexandria, VA: American Physical Therapy Association; 1993.
3. Reese NB. *Muscle and Sensory Testing.* 2nd ed. Philadephia, PA: WB Saunders, Co; 2005.
4. Shaurbert K, Bohannon RW. Reliability of sit-to-stand test over dispersed test sessions. *Isokinetic and Exercise Science.* 2005;13:119-122.
5. Norkin CC, White DJ. *Measurement of Joint Motion: A Guide to Goniometry.* 3rd ed. Philadephia, PA: FA Davis; 2003.

## Chapter 8

# Writing the Assessment and the Plan

*Rebecca McKnight, PT, MS*

## Chapter Objectives

Upon completion of this chapter, the reader will be able to:

1. List the type of information that should be recorded in the assessment portion of a SOAP note.
2. Describe the relationship between the evaluation and the examination.
3. Discuss the two aspects of a physical therapy diagnosis and describe how both are integrated into the written documentation.
4. Describe the difference between a medical diagnosis and a physical therapy diagnosis.
5. Describe the importance of the assessment and plan in relationship to the clinical decision-making process.
6. Describe the importance of the assessment and plan in relationship to reimbursement.
7. Construct short- and long-term goals in the form of a behavioral objective that includes all pertinent information.
8. Organize given evaluation information into a properly structured assessment documentation.

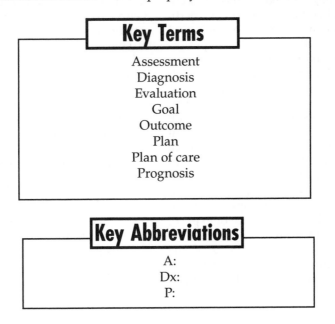

### Key Terms

Assessment
Diagnosis
Evaluation
Goal
Outcome
Plan
Plan of care
Prognosis

### Key Abbreviations

A:
Dx:
P:

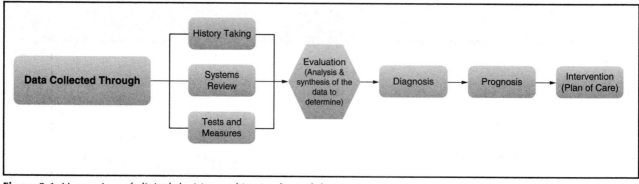

**Figure 8-1.** Linear view of clinical decision-making in physical therapy.

# Introduction

Following the examination, the physical therapist (PT) reviews the data collected (history, systems review, and tests and measures) and synthesizes the information to determine the physical therapy diagnosis, prognosis, and plan of care. According to *The Guide to Physical Therapist Practice*,[1] this clinical reasoning process is known as the *evaluation*. It is important to recognize the dynamic nature of the examination and evaluation processes. At first glance, the examination and evaluation appear to be linear in nature, meaning the examination points to the evaluation, which then leads to the diagnosis and prognosis (Figure 8-1). In reality, there is often interplay between the examination and the evaluation. *The Guide to Physical Therapist Practice* defines evaluation as, "A dynamic process in which the physical therapist makes clinical judgments based on data gathered during the examination."[1(p35)] Throughout the examination process, the therapist will make clinical judgments on various pieces of information. The PT then determines if further data needs to be gathered through a medical record documentation review, collaboration with other medical professionals, further subjective questioning of the patient or patient's family/caregiver, or performance of additional tests and measures. In his article "Clinical Reasoning in Manual Therapy," Jones[2] outlined the "cyclical character of the clinical reasoning process" and described the "hypothetico-deductive method" that therapists use during the evaluation process. Jones[2] further elaborated on the different characteristics of clinical reasoning between novice and expert clinicians. He ascribed greater efficiency in the expert's clinical reasoning to "a superior organization of knowledge and use of a combination of hypothetic-deductive reasoning and pattern recognition, or forward reasoning."[2] In either case (novice or expert), during the examination and evaluation process, the therapist will develop an initial hypothesis of the clinical problem(s) and proceed with the examination by choosing questions and tests that confirm or deny the working hypothesis. Each question or test will provide information that will feed back into the process "until sufficient information is obtained to make a diagnostic and management decision."[2] The therapist's clinical judgments and "management decisions" that occur during the evaluation process are documented within the assessment and plan sections of the SOAP note.

# Assessment and Plan

The assessment is often the most difficult section of the note to write, but is definitely the most important. In this section, the PT spells out his or her thought process by describing why skilled services are needed, in terms payers can understand. In addition, the PT identifies the relationship between the patient's impairments and his or her functional status, including activity limitations and participation restrictions. Also, it is within the assessment that the therapist can rationalize as to why a patient may progress faster or slower than expected. The "A" portion of the note is the section where the PT really describes both why the patient is in need of the service and how the patient will benefit from PT services.

In the assessment portion of an evaluative note, the therapist assigns clinical meaning, or value (evaluation) to the data collected during the examination process and documented within the subjective and objective sections of the SOAP note. Specifically, it is within the assessment section of the note that the therapist:

- Summarizes the patient's status
- Provides a plausible physical therapy diagnosis
- Spells out the relationship between impairments and function
- Identifies the patient's physical therapy problem(s)

Table 8-1

## Correlation Between the **Assessment** Portion of a SOAP Note and APTA's Patient/Client Management Model

| Patient/Client Management Model | SOAP Evaluative Note |
|---|---|
| **Examination** | |
| • History | Problem (Pr:) <br> Subjective (S:) |
| • Systems Review <br> • Tests and Measurements | Objective (O:) |
| **Evaluation** <br> **Diagnosis** <br> **Prognosis** | Assessment (A:) |
| **Intervention** | Plan (P:) |

- Delineates the need for skilled services
- Discusses the patient's other problems (medical, social, financial) that can impact the patient's physical functioning or participation with a plan of care (co-morbidities or complexities)
- Gives the prognosis in terms of reasonable, measurable goals
- Indicates the patient's potential to benefit from physical therapy interventions.

If the PT has determined during the examination and evaluation process that physical therapy services are not indicated, the therapist would document the rationale for this conclusion and provide any suggestions for alternate care that might be beneficial to the patient, eg, referral to a physician.

## What Type of Information Is It?

Information within the subjective portion of the note is information about the patient or the patient's condition as provided by the patient or other individuals associated with the patient. Information documented in the objective portion of the note is findings from observations or tests and measures directly gathered by the PT. Information found in the assessment portion of the note is the PT's professional interpretation of the data documented in the "S" and "O" sections. All evidence collected and documented during the examination should support conclusions and clinical judgments documented in the assessment. Therefore, any clinical impression provided within the assessment portion of the note must relate to data found within the subjective and/or objective findings. Elements of the Patient/Client Management Model documented within the assessment portion of a SOAP note include the physical therapy diagnosis and the

prognosis (which includes the plan of care) (Table 8-1; Also refer to Table 2-1).

### Summary Statement and Physical Therapy Diagnosis

A critical component of the assessment section is a brief summary of the patient, which includes the physical therapy diagnosis, need for skilled care, and an overview of any co-morbidities that may influence the outcome. Diagnosis is defined as, "both a process and a label."[1] Documentation of the physical therapy diagnosis should incorporate both aspects of this definition. "Diagnosis as a process includes integrating and evaluating the data obtained during the examination to describe the patient/client condition in terms that will guide the prognosis, the plan of care, and intervention strategies."[1] Within the evaluative note, the therapist should not only assign a diagnostic "label," but should also describe the rationale for the label by referring to the examination findings. As a component of documenting the diagnosis, the therapist should include clarification statements, summarizing the relationship between the body impairments and the patient's functional status such as activity limitations and participation restrictions that exist, or potential disabilities that may result if the impairments and functional limitations are not addressed appropriately.

When assigning a diagnostic label, it is recommended that the therapist utilize language consistent with a physical therapy diagnosis so as not to cause confusion (or conflict) with the medical diagnosis. As stated in *The Guide to Physical Therapist Practice*, "Diagnostic labels may be used to describe multiple dimensions of the patient/client, ranging from the most basic cellular level to the highest level of functioning—as a person in society. Although physicians typically use labels that identify disease, disorder, or condition at the level of the cell, tissue, organ, or system, physical therapists use labels that identify the impact of a condition on function at the level of the system (especially the movement system) and at the level of the whole person."[1(p37)] Appropriate diagnostic categories can be found in the preferred practice patterns as published in *The Guide to Physical Therapist Practice*. Practice patterns have been identified across four systems—musculoskeletal, neuromuscular, cardiovascular/pulmonary and integumetary—and are designed to inform the clinical reasoning process and guide the selection of intervention strategies (see Appendix D).

## PROBLEM LIST

A common component of the assessment is a list of specific physical therapy problems to be addressed during the episode of care. The actual formation of a problem list assists in goal writing and determination of appropriate interventions. When creating a problem list, the therapist should include any impairment in body structures or body functions, any functional or activity limitation, and any disability or participation restrictions identified during the examination and evaluation process that will be addressed within the plan of care. In the problem list, as within all physical therapy documentation, the focus should be on function. Impairments in body structure or function can be included, but clear connections between the impairments and function should be indicated.

## Prognosis and Plan of Care

As part of the assessment, the PT should include a statement of "the predicted optimal level of improvement in function and the amount of time needed to reach that level."[1] This is known as the *prognosis*. The prognosis is frequently recorded in the form of long-term, discharge, or outcome goals and includes a specific time frame for achievement and overall potential for achievement. In addition, as part of the prognosis, the PT will clearly outline a plan of care. A *plan of care* is defined as, "statements that specify the goals and outcomes, predicted level of optimal improvement, specific interventions to be used, and proposed duration and frequency of the interventions that are required to reach the goals and outcomes. The plan of care includes the anticipated discharge plans."[1] In keeping with the SOAP framework, specific goals, expected outcomes and level of optimal improvement are documented within the "A:" portion of the note, while the specific interventions, and the proposed duration and the frequency of interventions will be documented within the "P". As mentioned above, it is recommended the therapist include a summarizing statement related to the patient's potential (prognosis) also within the assessment section (refer to Table 8-1). Details of the expected outcomes, however, are documented as goal statements.

## DETERMINING THE PROGNOSIS

Determination of the patient's potential for recovery and the anticipated time for expected outcomes to be achieved is dependent upon a variety of factors. The most significant factor is the patient's medical diagnosis. For example, the expectations for recovery

---

### Example 1

A: 59 y.o. male s/p fall at work sustaining a (R) RTC tear, now 1 week s/p repair (ICD-9 840.4); PT diagnosis is impaired joint mobility, motor function, muscle performance and ROM 2° to connective tissue dysfunction (Pattern 4D). Impairments are limiting pt.'s ability to elevate arm overhead, reach overhead cabinets, perform normal home management tasks, or work activities as custodian. Skilled care needed to progress the patient safely per RTC protocol and for pt. education on limitations 2° to surgery. Pt. has no significant PMH influencing treatment and reports motivation to RTW.

PT Problems:

*Impairments*:

   a. Pain at rest and with activity

   b. Decreased ROM

   c. Decreased strength

   d. Healing surgical incision with eccymosis

*Functional Limitations (DASH score 55/100)*:

   a. Moderate to severe difficulty on ADLs

   b. Unable to elevate arm overhead

   c. Severe difficulty sleeping

   d. Unable to manage transportation needs

   e. Unable to work

   f. Unable to participate in recreational activities

---

of function of a minor musculoskeletal injury are significantly different than the expectation for recovery of a degenerative neuromuscular disorder. Additional factors the therapist will consider when determining the patient's prognosis include co-morbidities, general health condition, prior medical history, general demographic data (age, education level), surgical history, and social history. Perhaps as significant as the patient's medical condition is the patient's affective, or psychological and emotional status. The complex interaction of all the variables will have to be weighed by the PT. The therapist will determine an estimated prognosis. Revision of the prognosis can occur for multiple reasons throughout a patient's episode of care. Possible reasons for revising the prognosis include the onset of a new disease or injury, a change in the medical plan of care, a change in the patient's social situation, or a change in the patient's willingness to participate with aspects of the physical therapy plan of care. For example, a patient who is recovering from a surgical procedure may develop an infection, which will impact the healing process and lengthen the expected time for achieving the expected outcomes, or long-term goals. The PT will take this new medical diagnosis into consideration and revise the prognosis accordingly.

## WRITING GOALS

Goals or expected outcomes are clear statements of the "intended results" of the physical therapy interventions. Goal statements should be directed toward the physical therapy problems as identified in the problem list and should indicate the expected change that should occur through implementing the physical therapy plan of care. Goals can address changes in impairments, functional/activity restrictions, or disabilities/participation restrictions. However, goals written to address impairment-level problems should include clear language to describe how accomplishment will improve the patient's function. Goals must be stated in measurable terms to allow for outcomes assessment (the determination of the effectiveness of the intervention strategy and the patient's progress). Goals should also be time limited, or include a specific time frame for achievement.

---

## Example 2

Building on our prior example:

PT Problems:

*Impairments*:

   a. Pain at rest and with activity

   b. Decreased ROM

   c. Decreased strength

   d. Healing surgical incision with eccymosis

*Functional Limitations (DASH score 55/100)*:

   a. Moderate to severe difficulty on ADLs

   b. Unable to elevate arm overhead

   c. Severe difficulty sleeping

   d. Unable to manage transportation needs

   e. Unable to work

   f. Unable to participate in recreational activities

The patient demonstrates an excellent potential for full recovery and to meet PT goals as indicated by his high tolerance for pain, his high motivation level and his excellent general health. In 12 weeks, the pt. will demonstrate:

   a. No difficulty with ADLs

   b. No difficulty in elevating arm overhead to perform overhead activities

   c. No difficulty with sleeping

   d. Independence in managing transportation needs

   e. RTW without limitations

   f. Full participation in recreational activities

   g. Final DASH score <12

---

### Example 3

*Example Plan section*

**P:**    PT BID for neuromuscular reeducation, strengthening exercises, endurance activities, mobility training, and family education. Will assess pt's equipment needs for home use and facility acquisition of the
equipment. Pt. will require at minimum a wheelchair and a BSC. Prior to discharge recommend pt. &
pt's husband stay in the independence apartment to assess their ability to manage in a "home like"
environment. Anticipate continued therapy through home health services will be needed. If patient
demonstrates good recovery over her rehab stay may recommend an extension of her stay to work
toward greater independence.

Joe Jackson, DPT

---

*Instead of*:

In 12 weeks the pt. will have AROM (R) shoulder WNL.

*Use*:

In 12 weeks the pt. will have AROM (R) shoulder flexion 170° to enable reaching overhead and performing work duties.

Physical therapy goals should focus on an attribute or behavior of the patient instead of on the process or an activity. For instance, if a patient is receiving therapeutic exercises to improve quadriceps strength in the right leg, a goal written as a behavioral objective would focus on the attribute (the strength measurement to be achieved) rather than on the intervention activity (the therapeutic exercise).

*Instead of*:

In 4 weeks, the patient will perform strengthening exercises for the right quadriceps muscle.

*Use*:

In four weeks, the patient will demonstrate (R) quadriceps muscle strength 5/5 to improve ascending and descending stairs.

Physical therapy goals should also be written as behavioral objectives. A well-written behavioral objective is specific, measurable, and paints a very clear picture of the expected outcome and includes several parts. Many individuals learn the components of a behavioral objective by using the beginning of the alphabet as a guide. Here are the ABC's of a behavioral objective.

- "A" stands for *audience*. This is the individual who will be demonstrating the behavior or the attribute. For physical therapy goals, the "A" should be the patient or the patient's family member or caregiver. The "A" is not the therapist or another health care provider.

- "B" stands for *behavior*. The behavior is the action or attributes being performed or assessed. A behavior might be a functional task like walking or getting in or out of bed or it might be learned information like hip precautions. Or, a behavior might be a specific attribute the patient displays such as muscle strength, blood pressure, or pain.

- "C" stands for *condition*. This includes a description of the conditions under which the behavior is to be performed. Conditions could include the environmental setting in which the behavior will be performed or the presence or absence of assistive or adaptive equipment to be provided.

- "D" stands for *degree*. This is the degree of the attribute that should be demonstrated. This is a measurable term. A degree might be the specific muscle grade that is expected, the time it will take to complete a task, or the accuracy that is expected for a coordination test.

- "E" stands for *expected duration*. This is the amount of time that is expected for the outcome to be achieved. This can be stated in a number of days, weeks, months, or visits.

Another acronym that is often used to describe appropriately structured goals is *SMART*. SMART stands for specific, measurable, attainable, realistic and timely. This acronym incorporates many of the components as outlined in the ABC method, but it also highlights the concept of making sure the goals are attainable and realistic. When a clear expectation of the patient's prognosis is difficult to determine due to the complexity of the problems, the therapist should document this and set conservative goals. Reassessment throughout the episode of care should occur and revision of goals can occur as the patient's condition changes or becomes more clear.

### Long-Term Goals/Expected Outcomes

Long-term goals are statements of the patient's anticipated level of function by the end of an episode of care. Long-term goals can also be the outcome expectations for a particular setting. For example, a patient who is recovering from a cerebrovascular accident may receive physical therapy services on an acute rehab unit. The PT will set long-term goals related to the time the patient will be on that unit, while anticipating that the episode of physical therapy care will continue either on an outpatient basis or through home-health services. Long-term goals should relate directly to the identified problem list. Long-term goals can be written in such a way as to address more than one problem, but all problems should be related to at least one goal. Long-term goals are typically written for a time frame of weeks or months.

## SHORT-TERM GOALS

If there is a significant difference between the patient's current condition and the expected outcomes (long-term goals), the therapist should include short-term goals. Short-term goals can be seen as "bridge" goals between the patient's current status and the long-term expected outcomes. Short-term goals are desirable for several reasons. One reason is to help guide the decision-making process. As the patient progresses thorough the episode of care, short-term goals are used as landmarks or stepping stones to help the therapist determine if the patient is making the desired/expected progress within a reasonable amount of time. Without identifying short-term goals, it can be more difficult for the therapist to gauge if the patient is making satisfactory progress. Short-term goals also provide an excellent recording mechanism for third-party payers to demonstrate the patient's response to the physical therapy plan of care. Third-party payers demand documentation that interventions are indeed impacting the patient's problem(s). Short-term goals are a useful method to allow clear communication of the patient's progress. Finally, short-term goals provide a motivating factor for the patient. During a long-term rehabilitation process, patients can often become discouraged with what seems like little to no change from day to day. Short-term goals can provide small but realistic expectations for the patient to focus on and can be used to provide feedback for the patient related to his progress in therapy.

Each short-term goal should relate to at least one long-term goal. Within the documentation, there should be a clear link between the short-term goals, the long-term goals, and the physical therapy problems. In some situations, all physical therapy problems may not be addressed by a short-term goal. Likewise, a physical therapy problem may not be addressed early on in the rehabilitation process. For example, a patient who has had a transtibial amputation could be participating in physical therapy prior to receiving a prosthesis. A long-term goal should be included regarding the expectations for the patient to ambulate with a prosthetic device; however, if the prosthetic limb is not available during the early stages of rehabilitation, a short-term goal would not be included in the initial documentation.

## Importance of Documenting the Assessment

As stated in Chapter 2, appropriate documentation is required in order to meet ethical and legal standards and to communicate with reimbursement bodies like Medicare and Medicaid. It is within the assessment section of the SOAP note that the therapist is able to document the patient's need for physical therapy services by showing that the recommended plan of care is medically necessary and requires the skills of a PT or a PTA. Documentation of the prognosis through the establishment of clearly written behavioral objectives provides clearly identified expectations for assessment of the patient's progress.

## How to Document the Assessment

When documenting the evaluation in the assessment section, it is important to be specific and avoid general or vague statements. The PT should clearly communicate why skilled services are needed. How interventions will specifically address the identified problems and lead to changes in the patient's status should also be described.

### Structure

As with the subjective and objective sections, an important consideration for writing the assessment is to use a structure that is logical and allows reviewers to locate pertinent data easily. Typically, in the assessment section, the therapist will begin with a narrative, elaborating upon the findings and detailing the professional interpretation of the data. It is within this narrative that the therapist should include a brief summary of the patient, the physical therapy diagnosis (using a Practice Pattern from *The Guide to Physical Therapist Practice*), need for skilled care, and an overview of any co-morbidities that may influence the outcome.

Following the narrative, it is advisable to include a problem list. The list can be organized in any order. One common organization methods includes grouping problems into the categories of impairments, functional or activity limitations, or disabilities/participation restrictions. Also, prioritize the problem list beginning with the problem that requires the most attention. After the problem list, long-term goals or outcome expectations should be included. Typically, long-term goals are presented in a numbered list. The list is often preceded by a lead-in statement indicating the expected time frame in which the goals should be achieved and the patient's potential for achieving the goals.

After forming the list of long-term goals, the therapist should compare the list with the problem list to ensure that all identified physical therapy problems are addressed by at least one long-term goal. Finally, short-term goals can be documented. Short-term goals

## Example 4

**Patient**: D.W.

**A:**    This 68 y.o. obese female demonstrates very severe functional disabilities from a brainstem CVA. PT diagnosis impaired motor function and sensory integrity associated with a non-progressive disorder of the CNS – acquired as an adult (Pattern 5D) Impairments are limiting the pt. from performing any ADL independently, pt. also with difficulty performing self care tasks including feeding self, combing hair and washing her face. Pt. is motivated and pleasant to work with.  Due to the severe deficits prognosis for significant recovery is poor however the pt. and her husband want to try to get the pt. back home. A trial of structured aggressive therapy is indicated to see how much functional return is possible for this pt. and to educate her husband on how to provide any necessary care.

Problem List:

*Impairments*:

    a.  Decreased strength in extremities (R) > (L).

    b.  Decreased coordination (L) UE & LE.

    c.  Impaired balance reactions.

*Functional Limitations*:

    a.  Severe difficulty with all ADLs

    b.  Unable to perform housekeeping activities

    c.  Unable to participate in social activities

<u>STGs</u>: Within 2 weeks the pt. will display:

1.  Mod (A) for bedmobility and supine → sit.

2.  Max (A) for bed → w/c slideboard transfer.

3.  Fair static and Fair- dynamic sitting balance to allow patient to be more independent with self care tasks and slideboard transfers.

4.  Increase strength ½ grade throughout to be able to achieve functional goals related to bedmobility and transfers.

5.  Improve coordination (L) UE & LE to be able to achieve functional goals and improve the patient's ability to perform self care activities.

<u>LTGs</u>: Within 4 weeks the pt. will display:

1.  Min (A) for bedmobility and supine → sit.

2.  Mod (A) for bed → w/c slideboard transfer.

3.  Fair+ static and Fair dynamic sitting balance to allow patient to be more independent with self care tasks and slideboard transfers..

4.  Increase strength 1 grade throughout to be able to achieve functional goals related to bed mobility and transfers.

5.  Improve coordination (L) UE & LE to be able to achieve functional goals and improve the patient's ability to perform self-care activities.

*Pt.'s husband will*:

6.  Safely assist pt. with bed mobility and all transfers.

are also typically presented in a list format with a lead-in statement to indicate the time frame for these goals to be achieved (Example 4).

# Plan

The final component of a SOAP note is the plan. The plan section of the SOAP note should include components of the plan of care detailing interventions to be provided as well as the proposed duration and frequency of the episode of care. An intervention is defined as "the purposeful interaction of the physical therapist with the patient/client and when appropriate with other individuals involved in patient/client care, using various physical therapy procedures and techniques to produce changes in the condition."[1(p680)] Therefore, the plan should clearly detail all aspects of recommended physical therapy interventions including: 1) coordination, communication, and documentation; 2) patient/client-related instructions; and 3) procedural interventions. Additionally, the plan should state when re-examination or re-evaluation will occur and should outline the anticipated discharge plans. Discharge plans may include transfer to another setting for further physical therapy services (eg, transfer from acute care physical therapy to physical therapy in a skilled nursing unit), discharge with a maintenance program, or discontinuation of services. Finally, the plan should include a list of any equipment or resources the patient will likely require upon the time of discharge (Table 8-2).

## Coordination, Communication, and Documentation

"Coordination is the working together of all parties involved with the patient/client."[1(p39)] As an autonomous practitioner, an important role of a PT is to collaborate with physicians, nurses, occupational therapists, and other health care providers. Often individuals confuse the concept of "autonomous," mistakenly thinking it means that the PT acts in a totally independent, "Lone Ranger" method. Rather, the concept of autonomous indicates that the PT is entirely responsible for all aspects of physical therapy care. In order to accomplish that task, the PT needs to collaborate with the other members of the health care team. The PT has a unique and important perspective to share with the team, while at the same time having a responsibility to realize the limitations of that view. Therefore, the PT must have a high regard for the information and perspectives provided by other health care providers. Documentation within the plan should therefore include any plans to consult with other care providers. For example, if during the examination process the therapist determines that the patient's medication regime is impacting the patient's responses negatively, the therapist will document a plan to discuss these issues with the physician.

Coordination of care is accomplished through communication and documentation.

## Patient/Client-Related Instructions

The importance of patient education within the practice of physical therapy cannot be overstated. It is through the educational process that the patient and the patient's family or caregiver are assisted in taking full and complete ownership of the patient's health and well-being. Helping the patient develop the knowledge, skills, and attitudinal framework necessary to manage his or her own health care concerns moves physical therapy toward helping others function independently. Patient-related instruction can encompass several different topics, including education about:

1. The pathology/disease process
2. The body structure or body function impairments
3. Functional limitations
4. How impairments and functional limitations impact the patient's participation within social roles
5. The physical therapy plan of care
6. General health issues such as the patient's need for a fitness program or information regarding appropriate nutrition
7. A home exercise program
8. Home or work modifications
9. Functional task training
10. Precautions or restrictions
11. Appropriate activity level based on the pathology.

The written plan should outline specific information that will be a focus of patient education. The plan should delineate specific education topics that will be addressed. For example, a patient who is recovering from a total hip arthroplasty will require targeted information related to hip arthroplasty precautions. Goals should be included that outline the expected outcome behavior that the patient will demonstrate related to the patient education.

## Procedural Interventions

Procedural interventions include techniques and procedures used by PTs and PTAs (as directed by the PT) designed to impact the patient's condition in effort to achieve the goals and outcomes. Procedural interventions are the activities that most people consider when the term "physical therapy" is used. Procedural interventions fall under nine categories as outlined in *The Guide to Physical Therapist Practice*:

1. Therapeutic exercise

| | |
|---|---|
| Table 8-2 | |
| *Correlation Between the **Plan** Portion of a SOAP Note and APTA's Patient/Client Management Model* | |

| Patient/Client Management Model | SOAP Evaluative Note |
|---|---|
| **Examination** | |
| • History | Problem (Pr:) Subjective (S:) |
| • Systems Review • Tests and Measurements | Objective (O:) |
| **Evaluation Diagnosis Prognosis** | Assessment (A:) |
| **Intervention** | Plan (P:) |
| | |

2. Functional training in self-care and home management

3. Functional training in work (job/school/play)

4. Manual therapy techniques

5. Prescription, application, and (as appropriate) fabrication of devices and equipment

6. Airway clearance techniques

7. Integumentary repair and protective techniques

8. Electrotherapeutic modalities

9. Physical agents and mechanical modalities

When outlining the procedural interventions that will be included, the PT should include enough detail to clearly outline how the intervention will be used, but this should not be written in a way that will require unnecessarily frequent updates to the plan of care. For example, the therapist might indicate that electrotherapeutic agents will be utilized to address pain, but specific parameters do not necessarily need to be indicated. This will allow the therapist to choose between different devices and alter the parameters without the necessity of updating the plan of care each time. Documentation of the plan of care should demonstrate the rationale for the interventions by indicating the linkage between the procedural interventions, the patient's physical therapy problems and the established goals.

## Structure

Typically, the plan is written in a narrative format. The plan should include the planned interventions and the recommended amount, frequency, and dura-

tion of physical therapy services (see Example 4). Specific interventions can also be documented in a numbered list. When writing the plan, the therapist will use phrases like "Will check…", "Will update…", "Will consult….", "Will increase….," "Will hold….," "Will initiate…..". In general, the plan should include anything the therapist is thinking about doing that relates to care of the patient. The plan serves as a reminder to the therapist for future sessions with the client, or it can provide a guide for another therapist or assistant who might be working with the patient.

---

**Example 5**

**P:**    PT BID for neuromuscular reeducation, strengthening exercises, endurance activities, mobility training and family education. Will assess pt's equipment needs for home use and facility acquisition of the equipment. Pt. will require at minimum a wheelchair and a BSC. Prior to discharge recommend pt. & pt's husband stay in the independence apartment to assess their ability to manage in a "home like" environment. Anticipate continued therapy through home health services will be needed. If patient demonstrates good recovery over her rehab stay may recommend an extension of her stay to work toward greater independence. Joe Jackson, DPT

*Physical therapy intervention categories compiled from* The Guide to Physical Therapist Practice

Coordination, Communication, Documentation

Patient/Client-Related Instruction

Procedural Interventions

- Therapeutic exercise
- Functional training in self-care and home management, including activities of daily living (ADL) and instrumental activities of daily living (IADL)
- Functional training in work (job/school/play), community, and leisure integration or reintegration, including IADL, work hardening, and work conditioning
- Manual therapy techniques, including mobilization/manipulation
- Prescription, application, and as appropriate fabrication of devices and equipment (assistive, adaptive, orthotic, protective, supportive, or prosthetic)
- Airway clearance techniques
- Integumentary repair and protective techniques
- Electrotherapeutic modalities
- Physical agents and mechanical modalities[1]

*Questions a PTA will ask when reviewing the assessment and plan portions of a SOAP note.*

- "What do I need to know to be able to effectively treat this patient?"
- "What equipment do I need to provide the intervention?"
- "What type of responses might cause me to decide not to initiate treatment or to stop treatment once it has started?"
- "What information needs to be included in the treatment/progress note?"

# How Does the Physical Therapist Assistant Utilize the A & P?

The diagnosis, prognosis, and plan of care, as found documented within the assessment and plan portions of the SOAP note, is of vital importance for the PTA. The PTA is restricted to providing interventions as directed by the PT and as outlined within the plan of care. As directed by the therapist, the assistant will reference the plan to determine specific interventions to perform. For example, if the therapist directs the assistant to work with a patient on functional mobility, the assistant will reference the plan to determine which specific activities need to be addressed. The assistant will also review the assessment section to understand the prognosis. This will help the assistant have appropriate, realistic expectations of the patient and anticipate the patient's responses to the interventions. If the patient is not responding according to expectations outlined within the evaluation, the assistant will bring this to the attention of the PT.

# Summary

At the onset of physical therapy services, it is imperative that documentation clearly outlines the findings from the examination and evaluation and includes a detailed description of the plan of care. The SOAP note is a common documentation format that can be used for this initial examination and evaluation process. The SOAP format outlines the findings from the examination in the subjective and objective sections and details the evaluation, diagnosis and prognosis within the assessment and plan sections. The initial documentation provides the format and foundational information upon which all future physical therapy sessions are based. All future documentation should refer to the structure and information provided within the initial note.

# Review Questions

1. What type of information is found within the assessment and plan portions of the SOAP note?

2. Describe the relationship between the examination and the evaluation.

3. Describe the relationship between the diagnosis, prognosis, and the plan of care.

4. Differentiate between a linear clinical decision-making model and a dynamic clinical decision-making model. Which model best describes the process that should be used within the physical therapy evaluative process?

5. List and describe the components of a well-written behavioral objective.

6. How does the PTA use the information documented in the assessment and plan sections of a SOAP note? How can the therapist structure the note to enhance the PT/PTA relationship?

7. Outline an appropriate structure for the documentation of the assessment and plan sections of a SOAP note.

# Application Exercises

1. Read the following goals and identify the ABC's of a behavioral objective. Also identify what components are missing. Determine if the goal addresses an impairment, a functional/activity limitation, or a disability/participation restriction.

a. STG: Decrease turgor and fibrosing by 50% (to a 7 cm x 15 cm area) within 4-6 visits.

b. STG: Decrease girth of (R) ankle to within 1 cm of (L) (ctr heel and sinus tarsus) in 3 visits

c. LTG: Pt. will demonstrate mastery of pacing and other overuse reduction strategies to allow him to return to work.

d. STG: Decrease pain to 3/10 during movement.

e. LTG: Patient will display normal gait pattern.

f. LTG: 4-6 wks; Pt. will be (I) w/ bed mobility & transfer including sup → sit, w/c → bed no sliding board and w/c → floor.

g. LTG: 4-6 wks; Pt. will be (I) w/ w/c mobility on level surfaces, ↑↓ curbs, and on uneven surfaces.

h. STG: The patient will verbalize 3/3 hip precautions without verbal prompts.

i. LTG: In 8 wks the patient will participate in a community outing with only min (A) of 1.

j. STG: The wound will have an area of 2 cm by 2 cm with 1 cm depth.

2. Given the following information from an examination, write a short-term goal if the expectation is that the patient will improve.

a. Strength: 5/5 throughout (B) LE's except (R) quadriceps 4/5 2° pain and (R) hamstrings 4/5 2° disuse.

b. 
| ROM | L | R |
| --- | --- | --- |
| DF | 0-20 | -5 |
| PF | 0-40 | 5 to 10 |

c. Mobility: Bed mobility rolling w/ mod (A) and frequent V/C's for sequencing and set up.

d. Transfers: bed/mat → w/c w/ max (A) of 1-2, dependent w/ all set up

e. Gait: Pt. ambulated 50' w/ SBQC and min-mod (A). Pt. displayed ataxia, motor planning and motor sequencing deficits.

## Example 6

Assessment:

Problem List:
1. Knee pain
2. Limited ROM and muscle length
3. Limited strength
4. Gait disturbance

STG's: 2 weeks
1. Decrease pain
2. Increase strength by one full grade
3. Increase AROM, PROM, and hamstring length by 20° and gastroc 10°
4. WNL gait pattern

LTG's: Resume maximum function of the (L) knee.

Plan: Continue physical therapy three times a week for ROM and strengthening exercises and gait training

3. Review the following information, and using *The Guide to Physical Therapist Practice*, identify an appropriate practice pattern that matches the description given.

a. The patient was a self referral. The patient's primary complaint is back pain. The patient demonstrates a flattening of the lumbar spine, increased kyphosis of the thoracic spine, a forward head and rounded shoulder posturing.

b. The patient underwent an ORIF for a hip fracture. The patient has pain, decreased range of motion, decreased strength and decreased mobility.

c. The patient is 7 years old and has a diagnosis of cerebral palsy. The patient demonstrates delayed motor development, abnormal postural reflex responses, difficulties with communication and delayed cognitive development.

d. This client participated in a community outreach health risk appraisal held at a local community center. The individual denied any history of medical problems other than hypertension. The individual reported a maternal history of stroke and a paternal history of heart disease. The patient was mildly obese.

e. This patient sustained burns to both hands while burning leaves in his yard. The burns were partial thickness burns.

4. Review the assessment and plan sections of the note as found in Example 6. Critique the note utilizing the following questions as a guideline.

a. Does the note provide a physical therapy diagnosis?

b. Does the note clearly demonstrate the clinical decision-making process?

c. Does the note draw correlations between information about body structure and body function impairments and functional/activity limitation or disabilities/participation restrictions?

d. Does the note clearly demonstrate the relationship between the problem list, the goals, and the interventions?

e. Are the interventions clearly detailed to guide the physical therapy process?

5. Using the examination information from question 9 in Chapter 6 and question 5 in Chapter 7, write an appropriate assessment and plan.

# References

1. American Physical Therapy Association. *The Guide to Physical Therapist Practice*. Alexandria, VA: APTA; 2001.

2. Jones MA. Clinical reasoning in manual therapy. *Physical Therapy*. 1992(72):43-52.

## Chapter 9

# Interim and Discharge Notes

*Rebecca McKnight, PT, MS*

## Chapter Objectives

Upon completion of this chapter, the reader will be able to:
1. Describe types of documentation that occur across the continuum of care.
2. Discuss the roles of the physical therapist and the physical therapist assistant in relationship to documentation of interim notes, discharge summaries, and letters to a physician.
3. Differentiate between a treatment note and a progress note.
4. Identify factors that would indicate the need for a re-examination.
5. Discuss the relationship between the exam/evaluation note, interim notes (including re-exam/re-evaluation notes), and the discharge summary.
6. Discuss the positive and negative aspects of using forms and templates.
7. Discuss the positive and negative aspects of dictation/transcription.
8. Examine the positive and negative aspects of computerized documentation.

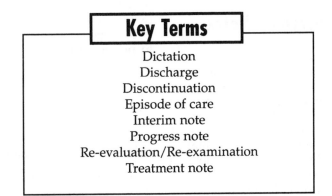

**Key Terms**

Dictation
Discharge
Discontinuation
Episode of care
Interim note
Progress note
Re-evaluation/Re-examination
Treatment note

# Introduction

As introduced in Chapter 2, documentation of physical therapy services should occur over the continuum of the patient's episode of care. Documentation of physical therapy services begins at the time of the initial examination and evaluation and continues with documentation of every visit/encounter via interim notes. Documentation is finalized at the summation of care, with a discharge summary. Interim notes can be treatment or daily notes, progress notes, re-examination/re-evaluation documentation, or a letter to a physician or case manager. The initial evaluation, any re-examination/re-evaluation, and the discharge summary should be written by the physical therapist. Treatment or daily notes and progress notes should be written by the clinician providing the intervention whether that is the physical therapist or physical therapist assistant.

The entire physical therapy record should clearly describe: 1) the patient's condition, or pathology, 2) impairments in body structures and body functions, 3) functional or activity limitations and participation restrictions that have been identified through appropriate tests and measurements, 4) the physical therapist's clinical reasoning and rationale, 5) anticipated goals and expected outcomes, 6) interventions provided, including patient education, communication with other disciplines, and specific procedural interventions, and 7) the final outcome, or result of the intervention. In order to demonstrate continuity of care being provided, each interim note should refer to the initial exam/evaluation documentation. Connecting interim notes to the initial documentation helps to demonstrate the clinical reasoning behind the plan the care. On the other hand, it is also important that each interim note include enough detail to support the interventions provided that day without the need to read the entire record (Table 9-1).

# Treatment Notes/Daily Notes

APTA's *Guidelines for Physical Therapy Documentation* indicate that documentation is required for every patient visit/encounter.[1] The primary purposes of a treatment or daily note are to document what occurred during that session or on that day in relation to the patient's physical therapy services and to support the billing codes that were used. Documentation of the patient visit should include the following elements: 1) subjective reports from the patient, 2) specific interventions provided during the session that are consistent with what was billed, 3) any equipment or written instruction provided to the patient, 4) the patient's response to the interventions provided including objective improvements made, 5) any factor leading to a modification of the plan of care, and 6)

any communication or collaboration with other health providers regarding the patient's care.[1(p686)]

To ease time constraints and facilitate consistency between clinicians, interventions are often documented through the use of standard forms, checklists, flow sheets, or graphs. Use of standardized paperwork will be discussed later in this chapter.

# Progress Notes

Progress notes are similar to treatment or daily notes and should include the information as outlined above. However, the focus of the progress note is not only to report the activities of a session but also to summarize the patient's response to physical therapy services that have been received. In a progress note, there should be a clear statement related to the patient's progress (positive or negative) toward the stated goals and outcome expectations. The frequency in which progress note are written is dependent upon the patient's rate of progress, the frequency of therapy sessions, the setting in which physical therapy is being provided, policies and procedures of the clinic/organization, and requirements by regulating agencies and third-party payers. For example, in an outpatient setting, CMS requires a progress note, or report every ten treatment sessions or every 30 days, whichever is less.[2] In general, progress notes should be written more often when the patient's progress toward the stated goals occurs rapidly. In practice areas that are not bound by policy or regulation to a particular time frame, progress note frequency should mirror the time frame as established with the goals. In some situations, each treatment note will be a progress note. For example, within an acute care setting when a patient who is recovering from a surgical procedure and significant improvements can be seen on a daily basis, a progress note should be written daily to demonstrate the patient's progress within the plan of care. Alternatively, within a long-term care setting (when working with a patient with complex medical issues who is expected to have a slow rate of response to physical therapy interventions) documentation of each session can be achieved through a treatment note and on a weekly or bi-weekly basis a progress note should be written to summarize the patient's overall response to the interventions and the patient's progress or lack thereof should be identified.

## Information Found in a Progress Note

Information found in a progress note should mirror the examination and evaluation and will include information from the patient or patient's family/caregiver, data collected through tests and measures and the physical therapist's (or physical therapist assistant's where allowable by law) clinical impressions.

Table 9-1

## Comparison of Information Found Within Each Section of a SOAP Note Between the Initial Evaluation and an Interim Note

| Initial Evaluation | | Interim Note |
|---|---|---|
| • Patient's chief complaint<br>• Medical diagnosis<br>• Physical therapy diagnosis<br>• Loss of function<br>• Any information gleaned from the medical record<br>  • Recent or past surgeries<br>  • Past conditions or diseases<br>  • Present conditions or diseases<br>  • Results of medical tests | Pr: | • Patient's chief complaint<br>• Medical diagnosis<br>• Physical therapy diagnosis<br>• Loss of function<br>• New test results |
| • Patient's current and past medical history<br>• Patient's symptoms or complaints<br>• Factors that cause the symptoms or complaints<br>• Patient's prior level of function<br>• Patient's lifestyle/occupation/societal roles<br>• Patient's goals | S: | • Patient's current status<br>• Patient's reaction to intervention<br>• New problems or new complaints<br>• Pertinent information not previously documented |
| • Information gathered through<br>  • Tests<br>  • Measures<br>  • Observation<br>• Interventions provided<br>  • Patient education<br>  • Procedural interventions<br>• Patient's response to interventions provided | O: | • Patient Status<br>  • Data collected through tests and measures<br>  • Patient's functional status<br>  • Observations<br>• Interventions provided<br>• Patient related instruction<br>• Procedural interventions |
| • Physical therapist's interpretation of the S: and O: data<br>• Identification of impairments and functional limitations<br>• Goals<br>• Physical therapy diagnosis<br>• Prognosis/rehabilitation potential<br>• Justification for goals/treatment plan<br>• Explanation of any difficulties with obtaining S: or O: data<br>• Suggestions for further testing, treatment or referrals | A: | • A summarization of the S&O<br>• Response to interventions<br>• Reference to how the patient is progressing toward the goals established in the plan of care |
| • Plan for intervention activities to occur<br>  • Collaboration/communication<br>  • Patient-related education<br>  • Procedural interventions<br>• Frequency/duration of therapy services<br>• Treatment progression<br>• Plans for further assessment or reassessment<br>• Equipment needs<br>• Referral to other services | P: | • What actions need to occur within areas of intervention<br>  • Communication/Collaboration<br>  • Patient-related instruction<br>  • Procedural interventions<br>• When the next session is scheduled<br>• Any equipment or information that needs to be ordered or prepared before the next session |

## Subjective (S:)

Information found within the subjective portion of a progress note should provide the patient's perspective as well as the perspective of others involved in the patient's care. Documentation should speak to the effectiveness of the treatment plan or need for alteration of the treatment plan. Documentation should include any comments from the patient or the patient's family member(s), caregiver(s) or significant other(s) that demonstrate: 1) the patient's status/progress, 2) the patient's reaction to interventions provided, or 3) new problems or complaints or any pertinent information not previously documented. Examples of information that should be included in the subjective section of a SOAP progress note are listed below.

*Patient's status*

- Pain rating and description (A 48 y/o male who is recovering from a total knee surgery was given a pain rating scale of 0 to 10. The patient currently rates his pain as 5/10 and describes the pain as a "pulling" pain)

- Patient's perception of symptoms (An 86 y/o female in a skilled nursing facility recovering from an exacerbation of COPD reports "I am feeling stronger")

- Patient's functional abilities (A 35 y/o female recovering from complications resulting from a radical mastectomy reports, "I was able to put the dishes into the cabinet last night for the first time since my surgery")

- Statements that demonstrate the patient's cognitive or emotional status. (An 84 y/o female recovering from an ORIF of a fractured femur. The patient has been a widow for several years and was living alone prior to the accident. During a physical therapy session the patient comments that her husband is waiting in her room to take her dancing)

- Comments related to accomplishment of goal/ outcomes. (You are working with a 32 y/o female who is recovering from a humeral fracture. One of her personal goals is to be able to care for her 10 month old infant. Today in the clinical she proudly reports "I was able to change the baby's diaper last night all by myself")

*Patient's reaction to interventions provided*

- Behavior of the patient's pain since the previous intervention. (A 52 y/o female is receiving therapy due to a diagnosis of adhesive capsulitis. The patient states that her pain level increased after her last therapy session when a new stretching activity was initiated but she reports the increase in pain only lasted about an hour and then the pain returned to its normal level)

- Comments that demonstrate if the intervention provided is effective (A 64 y/o male suffering from chronic cervical pain has received a trial of TENS. The patient reports no relief of pain symptoms with the TENS trial)

*New problem(s) or new complaint(s)*

- New pain complaints (A 77 y/o male patient is recovering from an elective THA. The patient had medical complications and was on bedrest longer than anticipated and his recovery has been delayed. As you begin working with him he comments that his heels have been very sore from lying on the bed so much)

*Pertinent information not previously documented*

- Medical history (You are working in an outpatient setting. You have been assisting with the care of a 48 y/o male who injured his back while moving. During his third visit, for the first time, the patient discloses that he had a hernia repair surgery 2 years ago)

- Environment: lifestyle, home situation, work, school (You have been assisting with the care of a 72 y/o man in a skilled nursing facility. He had a femur fracture and will be NWB for 6-8 weeks per the physician's report. The patient's goal is to return home where he lives alone. The patient reported in the examination that he has 4 steps without any railing to enter his home. As you are working with the patient during a subsequent session he reveals that his "steps" are nothing more than cinder blocks stacked on top of each other)

## Objective (O:)

Information found within the objective section of a progress note should include the verifiable evidence collected during data collection activities, as well as a clear description of the interventions that have been provided. It is important that the physical therapist or physical therapist assistant include enough details of the procedures performed (either tests and measures or interventions) so they could be reproduced by another clinician and to support the billing codes being used. Objective information documented in an interim or progress note falls into one of two categories: 1) patient status (changes in objective and measurable findings as they relate to the initial examination and the existing goals) and 2) interventions provided.

When documenting interventions the following information should be included: 1) Specific intervention provided (ie, patient education related to exercise, physical agent or functional training), 2) the intervention "dosage" (ie, number of repetitions, distance ambulated or time for a particular task), 3) equipment used (ie, TENS, 5 pound weight, standard walker), 4) equipment settings, 5) the specific body part/segment that received the intervention, 6) the patient's position if applicable, 7) the duration, frequency and rest breaks required, and 9) any specifics that would not be considered standard procedure. Examples of information that should be included in the objective section of a SOAP progress note are listed below.

*Patient status*

- Data collected. The results of all data collection techniques such as goniometry or manual muscle testing that provide a view into the patient's response to physical therapy interventions.
- Description of the patient's function. Ex. Description of the patient's ability to move around in bed.
- Observations about the patient. Any general observations that can not be categorized as data from a specific technique or a description of function. This may include information such as description of an open wound, description of patient's movement strategies or documentation of tenderness to palpation.

*Treatment provided*

- Communication and coordination (Discussion with nursing staff about the patient's pain medication schedule)
- Patient-related instruction (Education related to hip precautions with a patient who is recovering from a THA)
- Procedural interventions (Transfer and gait training, therapeutic exercise program, physical agents)

*Tips for documenting interventions*

- When documenting interventions provided include all information that is necessary to reproduce the activity.
    - What intervention was provided (Modality, exercise or gait training)
    - Amount of the intervention (Dosage, number of repetitions, or distance)
    - What equipment was used (TENS, 5# weight, standard walker)
    - Setting on equipment
    - Specific treatment area
    - Patient positioning

- Duration, frequency and rest beaks
- Anything that would not be considered standard practice

*Communication/Coordination*

- Physician
- Other health care practitioners (pharmacist, RN, OT, prosthetist)
- Administrators/case managers
- Phone conversations with any of the above

*Patient-related instruction*

- Therapeutic activity instruction (HEP)
- Precautions/restricted activity (Total hip precautions or lifting restrictions)
- Education related to disease process (What is a stroke?)
- Education related to physical therapy procedures (What is US and why is it used?)

*Procedural interventions*

Functional Training

- Types:
    - activities of daily living
    - assistive/adaptive devices
    - body mechanics
    - developmental activities
    - gait and locomotion training
    - prosthetics and orthotics
    - wheelchair management skills
- Include in documentation
    - Specific activity (bed to w/c transfers)
    - Assistive/adaptive devices used

*Infection Control Procedures*

- isolation or sterile techniques used (use of gown and gloves when assisting with ther ex)

*Manual Therapy Techniques*

- PROM
    - extremities/joints
    - number of repetitions
- Massage
    - location
    - type of massage
    - amount of time

*Physical Agents and Mechanical Agents*

- Types:
    - atermal agents
    - biofeedback

- compression therapies
- cryotherapy
- electrotherapeutic agents
- hydrotherapy
- superficial and deep thermal agents
- traction
- Include in documentation
  - physical or mechanical agent used (IFC)
  - pt. position
  - specific area treated
  - exact settings used
  - duration of treatment

*Therapeutic Exercise*

- Types:
- aerobic conditioning
- balance and coordination training
- conditioning and reconditioning activities
- posture awareness training
- range of motion exercises
- stretching exercises
- strengthening exercises
- Include in documentation:
- specific activity/exercises performed
- equipment used
- pt. position (if not clear by use of equipment)
- reps/duration

*Wound Management*

- Application and removal of dressings or agents
- type and amount of dressing used
- Precautions for dressing removal

*Equipment Provided* (theraband for HEP)

## Assessment (A:)

The assessment section of the interim SOAP note provides the therapist the opportunity to explain the relevance of the data documented within the subjective and objective portions of the note. It is within this section that the physical therapist will summarize the patient's progress, or lack thereof, towards the stated goals. This is accomplished by pointing to changes in the patient's status as evidenced by changes noted from data collected regarding impairments, functional or activity limitations, and/or disabilities or participation restrictions. When applicable, the therapist should indicate how interventions have led to the changes in the patient's status. Information in the assessment section should clearly describe the patient's response

to the intervention(s) provided and the patient's progress in reference to the goals established in the plan of care. This information should clearly demonstrate why continuation of skilled services is needed. The therapist should be concise but also specific. General phrases like "The patient tolerated the treatment well," or "The patient is progressing toward stated goals," should be avoided.[3] Every clinical impression should be supported by the evidence. Examples of information that should be included in the assessment section of a SOAP progress note are listed below.

*Patient's response to intervention*

- Change in pain level. (You are providing TENS application for pain control for a patient with chronic back pain with radicular symptoms. Prior to initiating intervention the pt. rates his pain as 7/10. After initiation of TENS trial the pt. rates his pain as 2/10.)
- Change in impairment. (You are assisting with the care of a patient who has lymphedema. You are using volumetric measurements to document amount of edema before and after intervention.)
- Change in functional status. (You are working in an outpatient clinic with a 32-year-old male who injured his back playing football with friends. When he enters the clinic his c/o pain and stiffness cause him to be unable to bend over to take off his shoes. After providing physical agents and appropriate therapeutic exercise, the patient is able to put on his shoes to leave the clinic.)

*Patient's progress toward goals*

- Whether a goal has been achieved.
- Progress toward a goal.
- No progress toward a goal.
- Decline in patient status.

## Plan (P:)

Within the plan section of a progress note, the physical therapist should outline any activities that are planned to address the patient's physical therapy problems. This includes documenting any collaboration or consultation planned with other health care providers, case managers or third party payers, any planned patient/client-related instruction, and all planned procedural interventions. The therapist should highlight any modifications to the previously stated plan. This provides the opportunity to emphasize the progressive nature of the physical therapy services. For example, the therapist can document that the plan is to progress the patient to a less supportive assistive device during gait, due to the patient's improved gait and balance responses. It is advised to restate the frequency of physical therapy sessions even if they are unchanged. Again, detailed and specific information is imperative. A general statement of, "Continue PT per plan of care," should be avoided. As stated above, each note should act as a stand-alone document. This type of entry would require a reviewer to search for the initial examination and evaluation documentation in order to determine what the plan of care is. Rather, the therapist should clearly state what activities will occur during upcoming sessions. Examples of information that should be included in the plan section of a SOAP progress note are listed below.

*Coordination/ Communication and Documentation*

- Consultation by the medical physician (the patient's orthostatic hypotension is impeding the patient's ability to participate in physical therapy and physical therapy interventions have been unsuccessful in overcoming the problem.)
- Consultation with other health care providers (consult with social services regarding discharge plans)

*Patient/Client-related instructions*

- Written instruction to provide (Will issue and instruct in HEP next session)
- Education regarding activity level/precautions (Will educate patient regarding hip precautions and car transfers)

*Procedural Interventions*

- Progression of treatment plan within established plan of care (increase resistance with therapeutic exercises)
- Modification of treatment plan within established plan of care (change from using a standard walker to using a wheeled walker due to the patient's continued problems with appropriate sequencing while using the standard walker)
- Equipment to be purchased (wheeled walker for home use)
- Activities to perform (focus on bed mobility training)

## Structure/Organization of Progress Note

The structure and organization of a SOAP progress note will be similar to the structure and organization of the examination/evaluation note. One difference between the initial note and a progress note is often seen in the subjective section. In the initial evaluative note, subjective data is often highly organized, utiliz-

ing subcategories. This high degree of structure is often not necessary in an interim note and it is infrequent that subheadings are utilized. While subheadings are usually not used, the therapist will still want to organize the subjective information by logically grouping similar information together. For example, all information related to the patient's pain (rating, description, and behavior) should be grouped together, while information related to home environment (distance needed to walk, steps to negotiate, type of flooring) should be grouped separately. Occasionally, the need will arise for many pieces of subjective data to be documented in a progress note. In this case, it is advisable to use subheadings in order to organize the information. Anytime subheadings are used (whether in the subjective or objective sections), it is recommended that the same subheading used in the initial examination be used in subsequent notes. This will assist in demonstrating the clinical decision-making process by helping to demonstrate a patient's response to interventions more clearly and promote continuity of care.

When documenting objective data, it is important to clearly differentiate between tests and measures data that have been collected to illustrate the patient's status and interventions that were provided. This is frequently accomplished by the utilization of tables of flow sheets for documentation of specific interventions. Alternatively, this can be accomplished by using subheadings, ie, Impairments:, Functional Status:, Coordination of Care:, Patient-Related Instruction:, and Procedural Interventions:.

## Documenting the Re-examination and Re-evaluation

*The Guide to Physical Therapist Practice* defines re-examination as "the process of performing selected test and measures after the initial examination to evaluate progress and to modify or redirect interventions."[1(p47)] Physical therapists will perform some aspects of examination and evaluation at each encounter with the patient. However, there will be various times throughout the episode of care when formal re-examinations/re-evaluations should occur. Re-examination should occur when there has been any change in the patient's status warranting a change in the plan of care. Re-examination will also occur as dictated by state law, facility policy or third-party payer requirements. Some third party payers will require a separate billing code for a physical therapy re-examination/re-evaluation; however, there are stipulations as to whether or not it will be reimbursed. For example, CMS requires that for reimbursement for a physical therapy re-examination/re-evaluation, there must have been a significant change in the patient's status warranting a change in the plan of care. It is important to be familiar with third-party payer reimbursement guidelines prior to using certain billing codes like "Physical Therapy Re-evaluation."

Documentation of a re-examination and re-evaluation should include the same elements as described for documentation of an initial examination and evaluation. The structure of the documentation should also follow the structure of the initial evaluation. An emphasis should be placed upon data that are new or different. The assessment section should clearly describe the changes that have occurred, goals that have been met, adaptations to the plan of care (goals, interventions, frequency or duration or care), and continued need for skilled services. All changes should be justified by evidence provided within the subjective and objective portions of the note.

## Discharge Summary

A discharge summary can occur at the completion of an episode of care or at the completion of care in one setting prior to transfer of services to another setting. In the "S:" section, the discharge summary will include comments from the patient/family regarding the present status, overall improvement, current pain scale or verbal rating scales, changes made to the home environment, changes in work status, or anything else reported that will support discontinuing the services.

The discharge summary also includes a summarization of the physical therapy services that have been provided for the patient's condition. The summary should also include a clear description of the patient's status at the time of discharge. The patient's status should be written objectively including data from relevant tests and measures. These tests and measures should be the same procedures and techniques that were used in the initial evaluation in order for comparison of the measurements to occur. Comparable data is required to make clinical judgments. Both the summary of interventions and patient status are written within the "O:" section of the discharge summary.

In the "A:" portion of the discharge summary, there should be a clear statement of whether the established goals were or were not meet. If the goals or outcome expectations were not met, a reason should be provided. A clearly stated rationale for discontinuation of service should also be documented. Examples of reasons for discontinuation of physical therapy include: the patient achieved all anticipated goals and expected outcomes; the patient/client, caregiver, or legal guardian declined to continue participation with the physical therapy plan of care; the patient/client became unable to continue participating with the plan of care due to medical or psychosocial complications; or the physical therapist determined physical therapy interventions would not provide any further benefit for the patient/client.[1]

A discharge summary should also clearly outline any discharge plan activities. Discharge plan activities might include referral to another physical therapist or physical therapy setting (eg, PT home health services), referral to another health care provider, recommendations for a home exercise or fitness/wellness program, suggestions for any future follow-up with a physical therapist, procurement of equipment, written instructions or training that needs to be provided to the patient or family/caregiver. As with the initial plan of care, all recommendations should be clearly justified by evidence. Evidence can be gleaned not only from the current patient status (measurements) but can be drawn from the physical therapy record in its entirety.

## Letters to Medical Physicians or Case Managers

Another type of interim documentation that is common in outpatient settings is a letter to a medical physician or case manager. As a professional courtesy, a physical therapist will provide a written update to a physician regarding the status of a patient who is under the care of both that physician and the physical therapist. This happens most often at the onset of physical therapy services following the initial examination and evaluation. However, it is also beneficial for the physical therapist to communicate to a patient's medical physician regarding physical therapy interventions provided even if the patient has sought physical therapy via direct access. Communicating in this way with the patient's medical physician helps to build mutual respect between health care providers and in turn helps to facilitate the patient's overall health care.

When writing a letter to a physician, the physical therapist should tailor the information to address the areas in which the physician is most concerned or interested. The physical therapist should share the physical therapy diagnosis, recommendations, and supporting evidence for the conclusions. A similar letter is often required by case managers. Again, information provided in this type of letter can be tailored to address the questions and concerns of the case manager. Any data referred to within a letter to a physician or a case manager and any professional reasoning or clinical conclusion should be drawn directly from the patient's physical therapy record. A copy of any such written communication should be kept in the patient's physical therapy record.

## Templates and Fill-In Forms

Templates and fill-in forms are frequently used by health care organizations. Each hospital, clinic or organization attempts to use efficient methods to facilitate documentation. Utilization of forms can help ease the burden of documentation and improve speed, efficiency and productivity. Forms and templates can also act as reminders to ensure that important aspects of patient care are not omitted and to help ensure that documentation requirements are fully met. Well designed forms and templates can facilitate accuracy and consistency in documentation. A disadvantage of forms and templates is that if not carefully designed, a form may not allow for documentation of all pertinent information.[4] It is important that the physical therapist (or physical therapist assistant) not be constrained by the limits of a form. A mechanism to include any information pertinent to the patient's status should exist. In APTA's Position on Authority for Physical Therapy Documentation HOD P06-00-2—05 after outlining general expectations regarding documentation it states that "Other notations or flow charts are considered a component of the documented record but do not meet the requirements of documentation in or of themselves."[5] Any form or template should be designed to provide an area for the physical therapist to clearly explain the clinical reasoning for PT services. Documentation templates for the initial examination and evaluation, treatment note, and progress reports can be found in Appendix C.

# Dictation

Dictation is verbal communication of information that is then transcribed by an individual or through computer software into written documentation. Transcription can occur immediately or information can be recorded for transcription at a later time. Dictation and transcription offer the benefit of flexibility allowing the physical therapist to include any pertinent information within the documentation. Although facilities utilizing dictation and transcription usually subscribe to a generalized structure for documentation (ie, SOAP format) typically, flexibility is allowed within that outline. Dictation can be a time-saver once a clinician becomes familiar with the activity, since it takes less time to speak information than to write it. An additional benefit to dictation and transcription is the documentation's readability, this leads to a reduction of error in clinical practice due to the inability to read the health care provider's handwriting. Drawbacks of dictation include the cost of transcription, transcription error, and the error due to the transcriptionist's inability to accurately hear or understand the clinician's voice; although, digital recorders are improving this area.

When dictating, it is important for the clinician to speak clearly and include any details that need to be included in the final document. For example, the clinician will need to verbalize if the information needs to be documented in a table format. In this instance, care must be taken to clearly describe how the table

should appear. After transcription has been complete, all dictated notes should be reviewed by the clinician to check for error. Errors should be corrected on the original form in the same manner as all error correction for patient care documentation.

# Computerized Documentation

Just as within our society, in general health care system activities are becoming more and more automated – especially in the area of computerized documentation. As stated by Eng[6] in *Tapping Technology: Computerizing Clinical Documentation*, movement toward computerization of clinical documentation and development of electronic health records is accelerating. This trend has been facilitated by several national initiatives.[6,7] In many health care facilities across the country, documentation no longer occurs with a pen and paper but rather is completed on a computer. Although computer-based documentation can range from basic word processing documents with fill-in form features, to complex computerized documentation software packages or web-based systems. The current trend is moving health care providers toward data systems that will support several organizational activities in an integrated format like billing, documentation, and scheduling. Vreeman et al[7] performed a systemized review of the current literature to determine the benefits and barriers to successful implementation of "electronic health records" within physical therapy practice settings. In their review, the authors found that published data on utilization of electronic health care records within physical therapy are limited. Upon review of 18 articles that met the author's specifications, the following benefits to utilization of electronic health records were identified: 1) improved reporting capabilities, 2) improved operational efficiency, 3) improved interdepartmental communication, 4) improved data accuracy, and 5) providing data for future research. Reporting capabilities were improved by the integration of clinical and administrative data, which decreased redundancy in data entry. With improved reporting capabilities, there were also improved mechanisms for service delivery and outcomes analyses. Improved efficiency of documentation was seen through decreased time required for data entry over hand entry and for dealing with reporting errors because of improved data accuracy. Interdepartmental communication was facilitated by improved readability of information over hand written information and by the ability for multiple users to access information simultaneously. These aspects helped facilitate improved clinical decision-making.

The authors also reported barriers to the implementation of utilizing electronic health care records. These barriers included: 1) the need to consider workflow or behavior modification, 2) the potential for software or hardware inadequacy, and 3) the initial and ongoing need for staff training. The authors discussed the fact that movement from a paper-based health care record to an electronic health care record is a system's change and therefore can have unforeseeable effects on workflow. Software and hardware inadequacies will vary from facility to facility and are a common side effect of implementing any computerization process. Careful consideration of the facility's expectations and the compatibility of the facility's current hardware and software can decrease these occurrences to some degree. Most of these problems are resolvable over time. Staff training is obviously greater during the implementation of a new system; however, updates and changes within the system will require ongoing training.[7]

One of the major benefits of computerized documentation is the standardization of terminologies and processes. Standardization can also lead to improved efficiency of a system and improved communication throughout an organization. Within this standardization, a level of flexibility for the needs of various departments can and should be achieved. Documentation software is designed to have flexibility for the development of templates that will match the needs of different settings and even for preferences of individual clinicians. Templates can be developed for examination and evaluations, daily/treatment notes, progress notes, discharge summaries, or physician letters. Documentation software can also have the capability of being integrated with reporting and billing software improving efficiency not just within documentation but also increasing efficiency and effectiveness of those processes. Of significant benefit is the ability to set prompts designed to remind the therapist when various processes need to occur such as re-examination or recertification.

Over the years, the sophistication of computerized software has grown, allowing databases to be developed that will provide the benefit of internal research for tracking visits, monitoring productivity, and analyzing outcomes data. These databases also improve data management to allow for clinical research which can provide a benefit to the profession at large. The development of web-based systems such as APTA's CONNECT allows subscribers the benefit of computerized documentation and also provides the opportunity for the development of a national database. The aggregate data can then be accessed by individual clinicians, facilities, and researchers providing each the ability to analyze trends in the provision of physical therapy services and in outcomes.[6-8]

When a facility considers moving from a paper-based record's system to a computerized system, a cost-benefit ratio must be considered. Cost consideration not only includes the financial outlay for the software or subscription, but also includes the cost in time associated with staff training and technical support. Additionally, in the rapidly changing market of computers, maintenance and upgrade costs for both the hardware and the software must be considered. Subscriptions to web-based systems will frequently include technical support related to software but technical support for the hardware components will also be required.

Security and confidentiality are additional considerations as is the need for "backing up" the information, and these policies and procedures must be in place. Some web-based systems have the advantage of including these considerations within a subscription, removing the responsibility from the facility. Any computerized documentation system must have in place a security method to ensure that only individuals who need access to the data can retrieve it. These expectations have been underscored by The Health Insurance Portability and Accountability Act (HIPPA). This act was created for the direct purpose of dealing with the handling of individually identifiable health information during electronic transmission. The HIPPAA legislation requires that facilities have in place policies and procedures for maintaining patient confidentiality.[9]

## Review Questions

1. List the different types of interim notes. What is the purpose of each?

2. How should a progress note be structured? How should the information relate to the initial evaluation.

3. List positive and negative aspects of using forms and templates.

4. List positive and negative aspects of dictation and transcription.

5. List positive and negative aspects of using computerized documentation.

6. What strategies can an organization utilize to facilitate implementing computerized documentation?

## Application Exercises

1. Research two computerized documentation packages. Compare the benefits of each package. What are the costs of the packages? What type of technical support is offered? What is the policy regarding upgrades of the system? What type of back up system is required? How user-friendly do the systems appear?

2. Interview two to three clinicians in your area about documentation formats used at their facilities. What do they like about the formats? What do they dislike about the formats? What do they think would be the ideal format?

3. Ask for copies of templates or forms used at two to three different clinics. Review and compare the forms. Do the forms provide adequate space to document all aspects of patient care including the therapist's clinical impression? Do the forms allow for ease of correlation of clinical findings with the clinical impressions? What are the positives and negatives of each form?

4. Write the following information in a more clear, concise manner, as it would appear in the medical record.

a. Upon arrival in the oupatient department for her follow-up visit, the patient indicated that she has been doing her HEP without any problems and that she feels that she is able to get in and out of bed easier.

b. You performed ultrasound to the dorsal aspect of the patient's right foot. You used 3 MHz at 50% duty cycle with the intensity set at 1.0 w/cm$^2$.

c. You instructed the patient to perform 10 repetitions of each exercise as part of her home exercise program. The exercises included ankle pumps, quadriceps setting, short arch quadriceps strengthening from 45° to 0°, and heel slides.

d. You are assisting a 18-year-old female who injured her knee playing basketball in walking with crutches. The patient walks in the hallway for 100' without you needing to help at all. When the patient attempts to walk up the stairs she tells you it scares her. You have to keep a hand on her to provide minimal stability for her to get up and down one flight of stairs.

e. You are working with a 42-year-old patient recovering from spinal meningitis. The patient currently needs moderate assistance to perform transfers to and from the wheelchair with a slideboard. The patient also requires occasional verbal cues for setting up the equipment for the transfer.

5. The following is an Initial Examination and Evaluation for a patient recently admitted to an in-patient rehab hospital. Use it to help you complete the two SOAP notes that follow.

---

**Date**: January 15, 2004

**Pr**: 72 year-old male 4 days s/p right BKA

**S**: <u>History</u>: Long history of chronic wounds on the right foot; recently developed osteomyelitis and gangrene and underwent short transtibial (BK) amputation. <u>C/C</u>: Phantom pain from the right foot, poor mobility, and decreased endurance. <u>L/S</u>: Pt. is retired coal minor. Lives alone in single-level house, with 2 steps at the entrance. Has never used an assistive device. Has been independent with all ADLs and IADLs prior to admission. PMH includes NIDDM, COPD, PVD, and HTN. Pt. is a non-smoker and non-drinker, although smoked 1 pack per day for 30 years. Quit when he was 50 y.o. Has one son living about 2 hours away who can assist on the weekends. <u>Pt's Goals</u>: Return to independent, active L/S, including driving. Wants to obtain a prosthetic device. <u>Communication</u>: Pt. communicates goals and needs without difficulty.

**O**: <u>AROM</u>: B UEs are WNL; Left LE is WNL; Right hip flexion 90°, extension 0°, abduction 40°, adduction 10°, knee flexion 90°, knee extension -10°. <u>PROM</u>: Right knee extension -5°. <u>Strength</u>: B UEs and Left LE are 4/5 throughout; Right LE not assessed 2° to acuity. <u>Sensation</u>: Left LE is intact to light touch, right residual limb demonstrates diminished light touch sensation around suture line. <u>Incision</u>: Horizontal incision line at distal aspect of the residual limb, no tension, complete closure, no drainage. <u>Pulses</u>: Popliteal artery 2+ bilaterally. Residual limb length is 2" from tibial tuberosity.

| Edema: | right | left |
|---|---|---|
| Knee joint | 22 cm | 20 cm |
| 2" below | 22.5 cm | 19 cm |
| 4"below | 23 cm | 18.5 cm |

<u>Balance</u>: Not impaired when standing in // bars. <u>Bed Mobility</u>: independent rolling and scooting. <u>Transfers</u>: supine ↔ sit with minimal assist x 1; sit ↔ stand with minimal assist x 1; toilet transfers performed with minimal assist x 1. <u>Gait</u>: Ambulated 10' x 1 in // bars with contact guard assist x 1 and 25' with standard walker with minimal assist x 1. Balance impaired when ambulating with walker 2° to decreased weight of right limb. <u>Wheelchair management</u>: Requires maximal assist for wheelchair management and can propel ~ 20' on level surfaces and then requires a rest break. <u>Endurance</u>: unable to ambulate more than 25' without shortness of breath. <u>Ther Ex</u>: 20 minutes of exercises including hip AROM: flexion, extension, abduction, and adduction; knee flexion and extension; hamstring stretching, and towel propping.

**A**: PT diagnosis: Impaired motor function, muscle performance, range of motion, gait, locomotion, and balance associated with amputation. Prognosis is good for anticipated goals and outcomes. Patient requiring skilled services for improving functional mobility including gait and transfer training with assistive devices 2° to amputation. Also required for preparing residual limb for prosthesis.

Problem List:

Impairments:

1) decreased ROM right LE; especially hip extension and knee extension

2) decreased strength right LE

3) decreased sensation

4) edema

5) incision present

6) impaired balance with walker

7) phantom pain

Functional Limitations:

1) decreased independence with ambulation

2) decreased independence with transfers

3) at risk for non-healing incision and skin abnormalities

4) impaired endurance

5) unable to drive

6) unable to perform necessary IADLs (grocery shopping, going to bank, etc)

7) wants to return to active L/S using a prosthetic device

Anticipated goals and expected outcomes:

After 8 weeks pt will:

1) Demonstrate full A/PROM in the right LE with no contractures—necessary for normal prosthetic ambulation

2) Right LE strength 4/5 also to allow normal prosthetic ambulation

3) Be independent with skin care and monitoring skin with use of prosthesis

4) Demonstrate 100% healing of his incision

5) 50% reduction in c/o phantom pain

6) Ambulate 100′ with walker independently

7) Ambulate 150′ independently with prosthesis and least restrictive assistive device

8) Transfer in/out of bed independently and perform sit ↔ stand independently

9) Obtain driving assessment

10) Participate in a community outing with only minimal assist x 1

**P:**    See pt. for 1 hour bid for ~ 8 weeks to work on the above through active and passive exercise, endurance training, gait and transfer training, pain modulation, balance, and pt. education. The patient is motivated and agrees with the above plan.

Betty Bopp, PT

a. The patient is now two weeks s/p right transtibial amputation. He is continuing to complain of phantom pain and sensation from the right foot. It resolves if he "squeezes" his residual limb. You are planning to attend a team conference for him on the following day, so you decide to take some objective measurements. Right AROM is: hip flexion 120°, extension 5°, abduction 40°, adduction 10°, knee flexion 130°, knee extension -5°. PROM: Right knee extension 0°. Strength: Right LE hip flexion 4/5, extension holds against moderate resistance in side lying position, abduction holds against moderate resistance in side lying position; knee extension holds against minimal resistance in seated position; knee flexion holds against moderate resistance in side lying position. The patient can not lay prone due to pulmonary problems and difficulty breathing when in this position. The incision is healing well. There is no drainage and no s/s of infection. It is moderately adhered to the underlying tissue and hypersensitive to pressure. Residual limb girth is 20 at the knee joint, 21 cm 2" below, and 20 cm 4" below. The patient can move and transfer in and out of bed independently to a bedside commode or chair. He can manage the wheelchair parts with verbal cueing. He propels the wheelchair 50' independently on level surfaces and carpet and then requires a rest. He can ambulate75' with a standard walker with supervision x 1 and his balance is good. You spent the next 15 minutes on patient education and exercise.

b. The patient is now seven weeks s/p right transtibial amputation. He is continuing to complain of phantom pain and sensation from the right foot occasionally, but it has decreased by about 75%. He has had a temporary prosthesis for about 2 days. Right AROM is: hip flexion 120°, extension 10°, abduction 40°, adduction 10°, knee flexion 130°, knee extension 0°. Strength: Right LE hip flexion 4/5, extension holds against moderate resistance in side lying position, abduction holds against moderate resistance in side lying position; knee extension holds against moderate resistance in seated position; knee flexion holds against maximum resistance in side lying position. The incision is not adhered to the underlying tissue and sensitivity has subsided. Residual limb girth is 20 at the knee joint, 19 cm 2" below, and 19 cm 4" below. He is independent with all wheelchair parts and transfer. He propels the wheelchair 500' independently on level surfaces and carpet. He can ambulate 150' with axillary crutches with supervision x 1 and good balance without the prosthesis. You spent the next 30 minutes on prosthetic training. He requires minimal assist to don and doff the socket and secure the supracondylar cuff suspension. He ambulates 50' with the prosthesis on and with axillary crutches with minimal assist for advancing the prosthesis. He is ambulating with an abducted gait on the prosthetic side. You spend 10 minutes educating the patient on skin precautions after removing the prosthesis and 15 minutes on exercises.

6. The following is an Initial Examination and Evaluation for a patient recently admitted to an in-patient rehab hospital. Use it to help you complete the following two SOAP notes.

a. You are working with a 67 y/o patient who suffered a (L) CVA. Today the patient states

---

## Initial Examination and Evaluation

**Pr:**  (L) CVA, (R) hemiparesis

Hx:  This 67-y/o male was admitted to the acute care 08-08-88 due to sudden weakness in his (R) UE & LE and slurred speech. Pt's PMH includes NIDDM, CABG x 2 07-05-85.  No other pertinent medical history.

**S:**  c/o: Inability to move around like he use to. Weakness in (R)LE & UE  Prior level of function:  (I) c̄ all ADL's and gait s̄ assistive device. Active; worked in his woodshop, yard and garden. Pt. is (R) handed dominant.  Home situation:  Lives c̄ wife who is healthy but is a small woman. Lives in two-level home c̄ 4 steps to enter.

**O:**  Observation: Noted 3+ pitting edema in (R) hand and forearm; pt. has tendency to keep (R)UE in dependent position.

Sensation: Pt. displays diminished light touch, deep pressure localization, proprioception & kinesthesia through the (R) UE & LE.

**Tone:**  Pt. displays diminished tone on (R) UE & LE to passive range, diminished patellar reflexes and absent Achilles reflex on (R)

**MMT:** (L) UE & LE; 5/5 throughout all musculature

(R) UE shoulder flex, ext, abd, MR&LR 2-/5; elbow flex 2+/5, ext 2/5; grip 1/5; (R) LE hip ext, add, IR 3+/5; flex, add, LR 2+/5; knee ext   3-/5, flex   2-/5; ankle df 0/5, pf 1/5.

**Mobility:**  Max (A) scooting ↑ in bed, Mod (A) scooting (R) & (L) in bed; SBA for safety and v/c when rolling to (R); max (A) rolling to (L)

**Transfers:**  Supine ↔ sit Max (A) from (R) side and Mod (A) from (L) side; sit ↔ stand max (A); stand pivot  w/c ↔ bed Max (A).

**Gait:** Not attempted at this time

**Balance:**  Fair static and Poor dynamic sitting balance; standing balance very poor.

**Endurance:** Fair; pt. tolerated 30 minute session requiring 1 minute rest breaks every 5-8 minutes.

**A:**    **PT Dx:** Impaired motor function and muscular performance due to CVA. Prognosis is good for goals as stated Skilled service needed to help patient improve strength and functional mobility including gait and transfers so that he can return home.

Problem List:

1. Edema in (R) UE
2. Decreased strength (R) UE & LE
3. Dependent bed mobility
4. Dependent transfers
5. Non ambulatory
6. Diminished balance
7. Diminished endurance

STGs:

1. Pt. will be able to demonstrate understanding of appropriate positioning for (R) UE.
2. Increase strength (R) UE & LE ½ grade throughout.
3. Pt. will require Mod (A) scooting ↑ in bed, Min (A) scooting (R) & (L) in bed; Mod (A) rolling to (L) and be (I) rolling to (R).
4. Pt. will require Mod (A) for supine ↔ sit from (R), Min (A) supine ↔ sit from (L), Mod (A) for sit ↔ stand and w/c ↔ bed transfers.
5. Pt. will stand c̄ Max (A) and quad cane for 1 minute.
6. Pt. will display fair static and fair-dynamic sitting balance and fair- static standing balance.
7. Pt. will display adequate endurance to tolerate a 30 minute therapy session only needing one 2 minute rest break.

LTGs:

1. Pt. will be (I) in (R) UE self care.
2. Increase strength (R) UE & LE 1 grade throughout.
3. Pt. will be (I) c̄ bed mobility including scooting  and  in bed and rolling to (R) or (L).
4. Pt. will be (I) c̄ sit ↔ stand and w/c ↔ bed transfers.
5. Pt. will ambulate 20' c̄ assistive device as indicated and Mod (A).
6. Pt. will display good static and dynamic sitting balance, fair + static and fair dynamic standing balance.
7. Pt. will display adequate endurance for a one hour session of therapy c̄ only one 5 minutes rest break.

he feels he is getting stronger and is looking forward to his first day pass to go home with his wife this weekend. The patient's wife states she is concerned about how they will manage in the long run. She says that their son and daughter-in-law are coming in from out of town to help out this weekend. In therapy today you worked on his bed mobility and transfers. He needed moderate assistance when scooting up and down in bed and scooting to the right. He needed minimal assistance when scooting to the left. He was able to roll to the right without any assistance and was safe with the activity. He required moderate assistance when rolling to the left. The patient still displays significant edema in his right hand and forearm and forgets to use his positioning devices in bed and in the wheelchair. He required minimal assistance when coming up from his left side. He requires minimal assistance when performing a sit to stand transfer and moderate assistance with a stand pivot transfer from the therapy mat into the wheelchair. You educated the patient's wife regarding his need for supervision and constant verbal cues to perform wheelchair set up and because he is impulsive and unsafe at times. Review the initial evaluative note so that you can make appropriate comparisons with his initial status. Be sure to include a summary of how is he progressing toward his goals and write an appropriate plan.

b.  One week later, the patient has returned from a weekend pass with his family. The family had considerable difficulty caring for the patient at home and they feel the home is not set up well for caring for him. The patient is upset at how difficult being at home was. He needs lots of extra encouragement today to participate in therapy. During his therapy session today the patient requires moderate to maximal assistance with rolling and scooting in bed and for supine to sit transfers when coming up from

his right side, and minimal assistance when coming up from his left side. He requires maximal assistance when performing a sit to stand transfer and moderate assistance with a modified stand pivot transfer from the therapy mat into the wheelchair. The patient needs moderate assistance and constant verbal cues to perform set up and is impulsive and a safety risk today more than usual due to his bad mood associated with his weekend. In your note, include a summary of how these findings compare with findings from the previous note and the initial evaluative note. Also briefly comment on the status if his goals and write an appropriate plan.

# References

1. American Physical Therapy Association. *The Guide to Physical Therapist Practice.* Alexandria, VA: APTA; 2001.
2. Centers for Medicare and Medicaid Services. Medicare Benefit Policy Manual. Centers for Medicare and Medicaid Services Web site; Internet-Only Manuals: 2006. Publication No. 100-02, Ch. 15-Section 220.
3. Clifton DW. "Tolerated treatment well" may no longer be tolerated. *PT—Magazine of Physical Therapy.* 1995;3(10):24.
4. Lewis DK. Do the write thing: document everything. *PT—Magazine of Physical Therapy.* 2002;10(7):30-34.
5. American Physical Therapy Association House of Delegates. Documentation authority for physical therapy services HOD P06-00-20-05. Available at: http://www.apta.org/AM/Template.cfm?Section=Home&CONTENTID=25443&TEMPLATE=/CM/HTMLDisplay.cfm. Accessed February 22, 2007.
6. Eng J. Tapping technology: computerizing clinical documentation. Available at: http://www.apta.org/AM/Template.cfm?Section=Publications&TEMPLATE=/CM/HTMLDisplay.cfm&CONTENTID=33355. Accessed January 28, 2007.
7. Vreeman DJ, Taggard SL, Rhine MD, Worrell TW. Evidence for electronic health record systems in physical therapy. *Phys Ther.* 2006;86(3):434-49.
8. Waldrop S. APTA Connect. *PT—Magazine of Physical Therapy.* 2007;
9. Ravitz KS. The HIPAA privacy final modified rule. *PT—Magazine of Physical Therapy.* 2002;November.

## Chapter 10

# Examining Your Patients' Outcomes

*Mia Erickson, PT, EdD, CHT, ATC*

## Chapter Objectives

Upon completion of this chapter, the reader will be able to:

1. Define outcome.
2. Recognize the importance of tracking outcomes for cohorts and individual patients.
3. List the contents of a discharge summary to facilitate outcomes data collection.
4. Differentiate between generic, disease-specific, and patient-specific outcomes instruments.
5. Differentiate between patient performance and patient self-report questionnaires.
6. Describe terminology and importance of reliability and validity.
7. Describe statistical measurements associated with responsiveness.
8. Realize the time- and cost-consuming nature and barriers associated with outcomes data collection.
9. Give practical suggestions for establishing an outcomes data collection process.

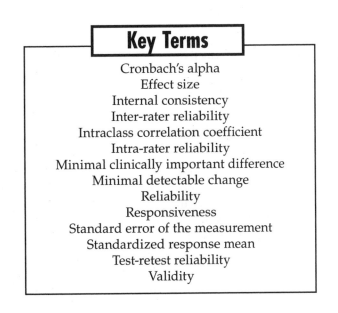

### Key Terms

Cronbach's alpha
Effect size
Internal consistency
Inter-rater reliability
Intraclass correlation coefficient
Intra-rater reliability
Minimal clinically important difference
Minimal detectable change
Reliability
Responsiveness
Standard error of the measurement
Standardized response mean
Test-retest reliability
Validity

## Key Abbreviations

ES
ICC
MCID
MDC
SEM
SRM

# Introduction

According to *The Guide to Physical Therapist Practice*, an *outcome* is the "impact," or end result of patient/client management.[1] An outcome can be a measure of the effectiveness of any physical therapy intervention(s), including: 1) procedural interventions (ie, modality, exercise program, etc.), 2) patient education (ie, body mechanics, ergonomics), or 3) coordination of care (ie, referral to another provider).

Also according to *The Guide*, the patient's outcome can include the effect(s) of the intervention(s) on aspects of disablement (ie, pathology, impairment, functional limitation, or disability), or on "risk reduction/prevention; health, wellness, and fitness; societal resources; or patient satisfaction."[1(p43)] In other words, a physical therapist (PT) wanting to measure outcomes can examine the effectiveness of any type of intervention on disablement, risk factor reduction, disease prevention, overall patient health/wellness, societal resources, or patient satisfaction.

*Outcomes measurement* is "a generic term used to describe the collection and reporting of information about an observed effect in relation to some care delivery process or health promotion activity."[2(p306)] Outcomes data collection has become increasingly more popular due to the need for proving intervention appropriateness, effectiveness, and efficiency to third-party payers. Additionally, Hart[3] reported that "payers cannot understand us when we attempt to communicate."[3(p1)] Using outcomes questionnaires or measures, we can provide a payer with a better description of how the injury or illness has affected the patient's day-to-day life in terms lay people understand. Hart[3] added that health-related quality of life (HRQL) outcomes tools consider the patient's perspective of his or her functional abilities and overall well-being, and they provide a powerful assessment of patient change during the time the treatment was provided.

Outcomes can be examined for cohorts, or groups of patients, or for individual patients.[2,4] Cohorts often include all patients undergoing a specific surgical procedure (eg, rotator cuff repair or total knee arthroplasty) or who have sustained a similar injury (eg, traumatic brain injury or spinal cord injury). Cohort outcomes are generally assessed by performing the same measurements on each group member at the same point in time. For example, a therapist examining the effectiveness of a balance and falls program might assess participants' balance and fall history prior to participation in the program, then again at 4, 8, and 12 weeks after beginning in the program.

Individual patient outcomes should be considered throughout the episode of care. First, during the initial evaluation, all PTs determine "an expected outcome" for every patient. This expected outcome is articulated through documenting outcome, or discharge, goals. Outcome goals or discharge goals may also be referred to as *long-term goals*. At each assessment and/or re-evaluation, the PT considers and documents whether the outcome goals have been met. This decision is made by comparing current and prior subjective and objective data. If goals are not being met, the PT determines and documents a reason they are not being met and rewrites goals as needed.

At the end of the episode of care, the PT summarizes whether or not the outcome goals have been met in a discharge summary. This discharge documentation should include the effects of any intervention (procedural, education, or coordination of care) on any of the following (Table 10-1):

- Pathology
- Impairments
- Functional limitation
- Disabilities
- Risk reduction or prevention
- Health, wellness, and fitness
- Societal resources
- Patient satisfaction[1]

Economic factors, such as time lost from work, lost wages, return-to-work status, number of visits, and total cost of treatment provided may also be included. PTs can also compare an individual's outcome to his or her other patients, other patients in the clinic, or to patient outcomes reported in the literature.

| Table 10-1 | |
| --- | --- |
| **Domains Addressed During Physical Therapy Interventions and Sample Documentation at Discharge** | |
| *Domains Addressed by Physical Therapy Intervention* | *Sample Documentation* |
| **If your intervention addresses...** | **Then you could document...** |
| Pathology | Pt. no longer showing signs or symptoms of complex regional pain syndrome |
| Impairment | AROM (L) shoulder is WNL in all planes and (=) to the (R)  Strength (L) elbow is 5/5 in all directions |
| Functional limitation | Pt. can ↑↓ stairs independently  Pt. can perform all transfers (I) |
| Disability | Pt. can participate in all school-related activities without limitation  Pt. is (I) and safe with unlimited community ambulation |
| Risk-reduction and prevention | Pt. demonstrates all lifting tasks with good body mechanics |
| Health, wellness, and fitness | Pt. is (I) with fitness program |
| Societal resources | Pt. is (I) in use of public transportation |
| Patient satisfaction | Pt. is pleased with her status and feels that she can discontinue outpatient PT |

## Selecting Outcomes Measurement Tools

Whether examining individual patient outcomes, or those of a specifically identified cohort, one of the first steps in implementing outcome measures is to determine what "measures" you plan to use. In doing so, you must determine what aspect of "health" or "effects of health-related problems" you want to measure, and then match the measurement tools appropriately.[4] For an abbreviated list of measurement tools, see Table 10-2. Another useful resource to aid in selecting measurement tools is *Physical Rehabilitation Outcomes Measures: A Guide to Enhanced Decision Making* by Finch et al.[4]

### Measuring Impairment

You might want to consider identifying impairments important to your patient population and determine an appropriate tool to measure the impairment. Simply put, if you are interested in examining range of shoulder motion in individuals with adhesive capsulitis, then goniometric measurements (when reliable) may be an appropriate outcome measure. On the other hand, consider a patient with lateral epicondylitis. These patients rarely have limited range of motion, so goniometric measurements may not be an appro-

*Selecting appropriate tools for outcomes data collection:*

1. Determine what aspects of health (or disablement) you want to measure.
2. Determine what measurements you want.
3. Determine what tools are available.
4. Examine psychometric properties of measurement tools.
5. Determine how to implement the tool:
    a. Administer
    b. Score
    c. Integrate into documentation
    d. Store and retrieve
    e. Report

priate outcome measure for these patients. In this latter group, it may be more appropriate to measure pain, either by a Numerical Pain Rating Scale or through a Visual Analog Scale. Other impairments often measured include strength, sensation, and balance. One problem with using impairments as outcomes variables is that payers may not be able to translate the technical language into functional improvements. In addition, some research suggests that reducing impairments does not correlate with improvement in

Table 10-2

## Abbreviated List of Measurement Tools

| Measurement Tools | Pathology/Purpose |
|---|---|
| Acute Care Index of Function (ACIF) | Acute neurological disorders |
| Alberta Infant Motor Scale (AIMS) | Pediatric motor development |
| APTA's Optimal | Mobility in adult outpatient population |
| Arthritis Impact Measurement Scale (AIMS2) | Arthritis |
| Asthma Quality of Life Questionnaires (AQLQ) | Asthma |
| Barthel Index (BI) | Personal care |
| Berg Balance Scale | Balance |
| Cardiac Health Profile | Cardiovascular disease |
| Cystic Fibrosis Questionnaire (CFQ) | Cystic fibrosis |
| Dallas Pain Questionnaire | Chronic spinal pain |
| Diabetes Impact Measurement Scale (DIMS) | Type 1 and Type 2 diabetes |
| Disability Rating Scale | Severe head trauma |
| Fatigue Impact Scale | Chronic disease |
| Fibromyalgia Impact Questionnaire | Fibromyalgia |
| Foot Function Index | Foot pain |
| Frail Elderly Functional Assessment | Frail elderly |
| Fugl-Meyer Assessment | CVA |
| Functional Independence Measure (FIM) | Variety |
| Functional Performance Inventory | Moderate to severe COPD |
| Functional Reach Test | Balance disorders |
| Gross Motor Performance Measure (GMPM) | Children with cerebral palsy |
| Gross Motor Function Measure (GMFM) | Pediatric |
| Harris Hip Scale | Hip arthritis |
| Multiple Sclerosis Quality of Life Index (MSQLI) | Multiple sclerosis |
| Neck Disability Index (NDI) | Neck disorders |
| Oswestry Low Back Pain Disability Questionnaire (ODQ) | Low back disorders |
| Parkinson's Disease Quality of Life (PDQL) | Parkinson's disease |
| Patient-Rated Wrist Evaluation (PRWE) | Wrist disorders |
| Peabody Development Motor Scales | Pediatric motor development |
| Pediatric Evaluation of Disability Index (PEDI) | Pediatric |
| Physical Disability Index (PDI) | Frail elderly |
| Roland-Morris Disability Questionnaire | Low-back pain |
| Short-Form Health Survey 12-Item (SF-12®) | Generic measure of perceived health |
| Short-Form Health Survey 36-Item (SF-36®) | Generic measure of perceived health |
| Sickness Impact Profile (SIP) | Variety with versions for nursing home residents |
| and Stroke | |
| Stroke Impact Scale | CVA |
| Therapeutic Associates Outcomes System (TAOS) | Variety of musculoskeletal disorders |
| Western Ontario and McMaster Universities | |
| Osteoarthritis Index (WOMAC) | Osteoarthritis |
| WeeFIM | Pediatric function |

For a more comprehensive list, see *The Interactive Guide to Physical Therapist Practice With Catalog of Tests and Measures* [CD-ROM]. Alexandria, VA: The American Physical Therapy Association.

function, quality of life, or participation in life roles or tasks. Therefore, you may want to consider collecting data on a patient's functional status, including his or her functioning abilities and disabilities.

## Measuring Function

### Generic vs. Specific Measures

Finch et al[4] described the use of both generic and specific tools for measuring function. Generic measures, or general-health status questionnaires, are not specific to any one pathology or diagnosis. Generic measures, like the Functional Independence Measure (FIM), are used to assess "overall" aspects of the individual's functional capacity, such as walking, transferring, bathing, dressing, etc. Generic measures are appropriate for both healthy and non-healthy populations and allow clinicians to assess physical function alone, or physical function combined with societal integration.[4] Some generic measures are also used to evaluate emotional response to injury and psychosocial issues through sub-scales. In addition to the FIM, other popular generic measurement tools include the Short-Form 36 Health Survey (SF-36), or its shortened counterpart, the SF-12, and the Sickness Impact Profile (SIP).

Specific measures of function include pathology-specific, body-part specific, and patient-specific measures. Pathology-specific measurement tools include items that are geared specifically to assess function and disability for individuals with a given pathology (disease), such as the Arthritis Impact Measurement Scales and the Fibromyalgia Impact Questionnaire (FIQ). In body part- or region-specific tools, like the Disabilities of the Arm, Shoulder, and Hand (DASH) Questionnaire, the Neck Disability Index (NDI), and the Oswestry Low Back Pain Questionnaire, patients are scored based on a set of predetermined tasks using the involved body part, eg, writing or turning a key on the DASH. Patient-specific measurement tools allow each patient to identify his or her own set of functional tasks he or she may be unable to perform due to the injury or illness. In using a patient-specific measure, the patient is not provided with a predetermined list of functional tasks. For example, the Patient-Specific Functional Scale (PSFS) requires the provider to ask the patient to identify three important activities that he or she is having difficulty with or is unable to perform due to the illness or injury. Then, the patient is asked to rate the level of difficulty on a scale of 0 to 10, with 0 indicating "unable to perform" and 10 being "able to perform at pre-injury level."[5]

Authors have identified strengths and weaknesses of both generic and specific measurement tools. First, generic health measures allow comparisons to be made across different patient cohorts and have relatively "good measurement properties."[4(p17)] Nevertheless, generic measures may mask functional problems specific to certain pathologies. Some patients seen in an outpatient orthopedic setting may score very high on generic health measures. For example, the patient

with lateral epicondylitis could potentially obtain a perfect score on the FIM, yet be unable to work due to pain and pain-induced weakness. Generic measurement tools may be "less sensitive to change than more specific measures"[4(p17)] and may "hide sensitive clinical changes."[3(p1)] This suggests that in patients initially scoring very high on a generic questionnaire, functional changes due to the interventions may not be identified on subsequent measurements.

Strengths of specific measurement tools have been identified. Specific tools measure functional problems often unique to a pathology or body part, and thus "capture" specific problems for that population. Questions are targeted at identifying disability due to a specific pathology, or injury to a body part, rather than evaluating general health-related quality of life. More specific functional tasks that appear on these types of questionnaires are generally not included in a generic tool. In addition, functional changes occurring as a result of an intervention may be seen more clearly using a specific tool rather than a generic quality of life questionnaire. Weaknesses of specific tools, however, have been described by Finch et al.[4] These authors reported that comparison of scores on specific tools is limited to patients with the same condition or problem of the same body part, eg, patients with rotator cuff syndrome or patients with acute low back pain. Finally, a specific measure may not capture general quality of life changes.[4] An additional problem with the patient-specific ratings is that comparisons across cohorts are limited because patients are likely to give different functional activities.

### Patient Performance vs. Self-Report

In performance-based outcomes measures, the patient is required to perform a set of functional tasks, such as the FIM. In using the FIM, the patient is assessed according to his or her ability to: 1) perform self-care skills (eg, feeding and dressing), 2) control bowel/bladder function, 3) transfer, 4) move (eg, gait and stair climbing), 5) communicate, and 6) interact socially, including memory and problem solving. Two problems with patient performance instruments are: 1) patients are aware they are being assessed and may alter performance, and 2) the time it takes to administer and score.

Function and disability assessments can also be "self-report." In self-report measures, the patient completes a questionnaire, rating his or her overall performance on a predetermined set of functional tasks. An example of a patient self-reported functional measure is the Oswestry Low Back Pain Questionnaire, often used to assess the functional status of patients with back pain. Other examples of self-reported questionnaires include the SF-36, the NDI, and the Patient-Rated Wrist Evaluation (PRWE). Two problems with patient self-report instruments are: 1) the self-report may be considered "subjective", and 2) a patient may over- or underestimate his or her function.

## Measurement Properties

### Reliability

*Reliability* is defined as the repeatability, or consistency, of an instrument or rater in measuring a variable.[6] One type of reliability is internal consistency. *Internal consistency* is a measurement of how "alike" individual items are in an instrument with multiple questions or tasks. The internal consistency value falls between 0 and 1 (Cronbach's α), and the closer the value is to 1, the higher the internal consistency.[4] Another type of reliability is *intra-rater reliability*. It is the ability of one rater to obtain the same score on multiple attempts. This is also known as *test-retest reliability*. *Inter-rater reliability* is the ability for multiple raters to obtain a consistent score on repeated attempts. Test-retest and inter-rater reliability measures are often provided in terms of an intraclass correlation coefficient (ICC) and/or the standard error of the measurement (SEM). Like Cronbach's α, ICC values range from 0 to 1, and the closer the value to 1, the better the reliability.[4]

The SEM is a quantification of the reliability, given in the same measurement units as the original measurement[4,7] (eg, the SEM for goniometry would be given in degrees). It is also described as the amount of error associated with a measurement tool.[8] The SEM value gives you the amount of error you would obtain in repeated testing of the same patient. Let's look at an example:

Two individuals measured knee range of motion on 80 patients following total knee arthroplasty. Their inter-rater reliability value, or ICC was equal to 0.75 and the SEM was 10 degrees. This means that the amount of error associated with goniometric measurements in these raters was 10 degrees. Repeated measurement of a participant in this study (i.e. before and after treatment) may be off as much as 10 degrees just due to error. This is important clinically because change scores before and after treatment that are less than 10 degrees may be due to error, rather than true change due to an intervention's effectiveness.

The SEM value is calculated in the following manner[8]:

$$\text{SEM} = \text{standard deviation} \times \sqrt{(1\text{-reliability coefficient})}$$

When estimating the SEM for a questionnaire with multiple items, administered at a single point in time (or for a one-time use), the reliability coefficient used is the Cronbach's α value[9]:

$$\text{SEM} = \text{standard deviation} \times \sqrt{(1\text{-Cronbach's } \alpha)}$$

However, when estimating the SEM for a change score, the test-retest reliability coefficient (ICC) is used to calculate the SEM[8,10]:

$$\text{SEM}_{\text{test-retest}} = \text{standard deviation}_{\text{baseline}} \times \sqrt{(1\text{-ICC})}$$

Let's look at a real example from the literature. Authors of a 2006 study published in *Physical Therapy* reported the SEM for measuring gait speed as measured on a GaitMat II.[11] In this study, the SEM for participant's normal gait speed was 0.04 m/s and 0.05 for faster speeds. We know that any change between baseline and post-intervention speed below the SEM may be indicative of measurement error, rather than true change due to treatment.

Let's apply these results to a patient in a clinical situation.

A patient's gait speed at the initial encounter was .82 m/s. After a 4-week physical therapy intervention program, the patient's gait speed was .85 m/s, a difference of 0.03m/s. In this case, yes, the patient has shown a change, and a clinician may be inclined to document there had been an improvement in gait speed. However, given the amount of error associated with the test, the change may be due to measurement error rather than true improvement in speed. Hence, a clinician should not conclude that the patient made significant progress.

After continuing the program for another 2 weeks, the patient's gait speed is reassessed. This time it is .92, a difference of .10 m/s. In this case, the clinician could conclude there has been a change outside the margin of error. This patient's progress would be recorded in the "A" portion of a SOAP note.

The SEM can help clinicians make decisions about which tools to use, as well as aid in making decisions with individual patients by comparing his or her measurement or change score with the SEM. Clinicians should become familiar with estimated reliability values and SEMs associated with tests and measures they use frequently, realizing that values are estimated by testing on a specific patient sample. Additionally, when data are not available for a specific patient population, a clinician may have to extrapolate from more generic data.[8]

### Validity

*Validity* is the degree that an instrument or rater measures the variable that it (or he) intends to measure. Like reliability, there are different types of validity. Additionally, there is a relationship between reliability and validity. Lohr[12] indicated, "the level of reliability dictates the highest degree of validity possible" and measures that are unreliable "can never be valid."(p39) But on the other hand, reliability does not ensure validity.[4]

Validity has traditionally been broken into four categories: face, content, construct, and criterion-related.[4,6] These have been defined by Portney and Watkins[6(p82)]:

1. *Face validity*: the extent to which an instrument measures what it is intended to measure.

2. *Content validity*: the extent to which individual items adequately "sample" the content defining the variable of interest.

3. *Construct validity*: the extent to which an instrument can measure an abstract concept, and the degree to which it reflects its theoretical components.

4. *Criterion-related validity*: the extent to which an outcome measure can be used as a substitute for the "gold standard" measurement.

Other types of validity described in the literature include *convergent validity*, or "the extent to which a measure's result is consistent with the result of another measure believed to be assessing the same attribute," and *discriminant validity*, "the extent to which a measure selectively assesses the attribute of interest rather than a general concept."[8(p169)] Another type of validity is *known-group validity*, which is "the extent to which a measure is capable of distinguishing distinct groups who are known to possess different levels of the attribute of interest."[8(p169)]

Portney and Watkins[6] suggested that many types of validity testing are needed when developing an instrument, and this is rarely accomplished in a single study. When examining a particular outcome instrument, the validity measurements of interest to you depend on how you intend to use the instrument.

## Clinical Utility

Finch et al[4] described four characteristics associated with a clinician's understanding of a patient's results for an outcome measure. The clinician considers: 1) normal values, or scores occurring within the normal population, although many measurement tools do not have established normative data; 2) the confidence interval for the patient's score, or how likely the score fell within a given range; 3) the minimal detectable change (MDC), or confidence of true change, rather than error; and 4) the minimal clinically important difference (MCID), or a value that represents an important, clinically significant change which the patient may also perceive as beneficial. Part of determining the clinical utility of an instrument requires researchers to estimate the MDC and MCID of outcomes measurement tools on various patient populations.

## MDC

An MDC at a 95% confidence level is calculated using the test-retest SEM value ($SEM_{test-retest}$) in the following manner[8]:

$$MDC_{95} = SEM_{test-retest} \times z\text{-value}_{95} \times \sqrt{2}$$
*or*
$$MDC_{95} = SEM_{test-retest} \times 1.96 \times \sqrt{2}$$

Authors examining psychometric properties of the Disabilities of the Arm, Hand, and Shoulder (DASH) Outcome Measure used this formula to calculate the MDC of the DASH at the 95% confidence level ($MDC_{95}$).[10] First, they calculated the test-retest SEM ($SEM_{test-retest}$) at the 95% confidence level using the ICC value (.96) and the baseline standard deviation (23.02) (Example 1). Second, they calculated the SEM at the 95% confidence level ($SEM_{95}$) as described above. Then, they multiplied the $SEM_{95}$ by the square root of two to determine the $MDC_{95}$:[10]

### Example 1

**Step One:**
$SEM_{test-retest}$ = standard deviation$_{baseline}$ x $\sqrt{(1\text{-}ICC)}$
$SEM_{test-retest}$ = (23.02 x $\sqrt{1\text{-}.96}$)
$SEM_{test-retest}$ = 4.6 DASH points

**Step Two:**
$SEM_{95}$ = SEM x z-value$_{95}$
$SEM_{95}$ = 4.6 x 1.96
$SEM_{95}$ = 9 DASH points

**Step Three:**
$MDC_{95}$ = $SEM_{95}$ x $\sqrt{2}$
$MDC_{95}$ = 9 x $\sqrt{2}$
$MDC_{95}$ = 12.75 DASH points

The MDC at the 90% confidence level ($MDC_{90}$) can also be obtained by substituting the associated z-value (1.65) for the z-value at 95% confidence level (1.96) (Example 2).

### Example 2

**Step One:**
$SEM_{test-retest}$ = standard deviation$_{baseline}$ x $\sqrt{(1\text{-}ICC)}$
$SEM_{test-retest}$ = (23.02 x $\sqrt{1\text{-}.96}$)
$SEM_{test-retest}$ = 4.6 DASH points

**Step Two:**
$SEM_{90}$ = SEM x z-value$_{90}$
$SEM_{90}$ = 4.6 x 1.65
$SEM_{90}$ = 7.6 DASH points

**Step Three:**
$MDC_{90}$ = $SEM_{90}$ x $\sqrt{2}$
$MDC_{90}$ = 7.6 x $\sqrt{2}$
$MDC_{90}$ = 10.7 DASH points

## MCID

The other estimate to determine an instrument's clinical utility is the MCID. Again, this is the change that would be significant to the patient. The "MDC and MCID values can be used by clinicians to assist in determining whether a patient has experienced a real and meaningful change."[11(p814)] MacDermid and Stratford[8] indicated that many factors influence the patient's perception of what is a clinically important difference, and the "magnitude of the clinically important difference is likely to vary depending on the circumstances."[8(p171)] They also indicated measurements to estimate the MCID "were still in their infancy."[8(p171)] However, Palombaro et al[11] recently listed several methods to estimate the MCID using: 1) patient self-report, 2) expert consensus, or 3) through calculation of the SEM or receiver operating characteristic (ROC) curve.

Let's go back to our example from the literature on gait speed.

Palombaro et al[11] used expert opinion and an ROC curve to estimate the MCID of gait speed. For this study, the authors reported the MCID was equal to 1.0 m/s. They indicated the MCID provided a "threshold for clinical meaningfulness with which to compare a gait speed change that is greater than measurement error (SEM)"[(p814)] and that would be meaningful to patients.[11] These authors indicated that a clinician working with a similar population may be able to apply these results when documenting changes in gait speed, realizing that the MCID is only an estimate.

Using outcomes measurement tools in goal writing requires clinicians to be familiar with properties of reliability, validity, clinical utility, and responsiveness. Understanding the MDC and MCID provides us with benchmarks to establish goals for a patient. Also, MacDermid and Stratford[8] indicated that knowing the score that coincides with a specific level of disability, or ability, allows the clinician to write specific goals integrating the measurement with a functional activity. They provided an example of a patient with rotator cuff disease (Initial DASH score = 44). In deciding goals for this patient, they knew from Beaton et al[10] that a score between 20-25 on the DASH coincided with a patient returning to work. They were also able to extrapolate from the literature that a MCID on the DASH is approximately 15. Therefore, they provided the following outcome goal for the patient[8]:

In 12 weeks, the patient will demonstrate an important change in his DASH score (> 15 points).

A 15 point reduction would result in a DASH score equal to 29, showing progress toward the score that coincides with return to work. Using the tool's measurement properties can be helpful in writing goals, justifying services, and demonstrating meaningful vs. non-meaningful changes in a patient's status. In an ideal world, data on measurement tools would be easily available to clinicians; however, this is usually not the case, and as mentioned previously, clinicians may have to extrapolate from more general research findings.[8]

More research is needed to determine how values such as SEM, MDC, and MCID can be generalized to patients in a clinical setting. Nevertheless, values identified in the literature provide a starting point for clinicians wanting to interpret test results and determine whether a meaningful change has occurred.

## Responsiveness

One additional measurement property of interest to clinicians is the instrument's sensitivity to change, or responsiveness. This is important because clinicians want to know if instruments can detect change occurring within a certain group of patients or not. Whereas MDC and MCID values help make decisions with individual patients, responsiveness helps to make decisions about which tool to use.

Methods used to calculate an instrument's responsiveness are the standardized response mean (SRM), effect size (ES), or standardized effect size.[9,13]

$$SRM = \frac{mean\ change\ scores\ (follow\text{-}up\text{--}initial\ scores)}{standard\ deviation\ of\ change\ scores}$$

$$ES = mean\ change\ scores\ (follow\text{-}up\text{--}initial\ scores)$$

*or*

$$SRD = \frac{mean\ change\ scores\ (follow\text{-}up-initial\ scores)}{standard\ deviation\ of\ initial\ scores}$$

Effect sizes greater than 0.80 indicate large effects, and an SRM value greater than 1.0 is a common value, or "threshold for establishing responsiveness."[13(p330)]

# Considerations for Collecting Outcomes Data

Regardless of whether you are studying individuals or cohorts, the focus of the outcomes measurement is on the recipient of care, not the provider.[2] For example, a PT measuring outcomes attempts to determine what changes took place in the patient. These changes could be measured in terms of functional performance, impairments, return to work status, return to independent living, or societal integration following a traumatic injury, to name a few. Measurements of provider actions, such as tracking patient education, are not true outcomes indicators.[2]

Data collected during outcomes measurement can be used for research, program evaluation, clinical guideline development, professional presentations, or management activities such as marketing, tracking performance for individual therapists or entire clinics, examining patient satisfaction, and for quality improvement. Lohr[12] reported that health status measures have potential for quality assessment, especially when the instruments are used repeatedly, so quality assessment is based on the patient's change over time rather than on a single evaluation. Nevertheless, she indicated that the longer the period of observation, the lower the connection between the outcomes and the care provided. In these instances, extraneous factors affecting both patients and providers begin weighing more heavily. Then it becomes more difficult to draw conclusions about specific providers and quality of care rendered.[12]

It is important to point out that extraneous patient and provider factors influence outcomes data. Patient factors such as disease progression, co-morbidities, co-interventions, adherence, motivation, socioeconomic status, educational level, and payer source may affect outcomes data either positively or negatively. Care provider and organizational factors such as documentation procedures, measurement variability between providers, differing intervention strategies, record-keeping, time allotment, data storage, and types of measurements selected to determine outcome can also influence data. In addition, Wakefield[14] reported, "from both a conceptual and methodological perspective, outcomes assessment must take into account all of the services received from all providers involved in the patient care process."[(pp111-112)] This is an important consideration in settings where the patient is receiving a multidisciplinary approach to treatment. For example, in inpatient rehabilitation, a patient may be receiving physical therapy, occupational therapy, speech therapy, neuropsychology, and nutritional services.

Ingersol[12] reported, "collecting and reporting bad data simply because it is available does nothing to aid in informed decision making or maximization of outcome effect."[(p302)] Clinicians starting to collect data for tracking outcomes should consider the multiple factors described above that influence their data. Lohr[12] reported that prior to establishing an outcomes measurement plan, you should determine: 1) its purpose, 2) the source of data, 3) the procedures and/or individual(s) responsible for data collection, and 4) an individual(s) responsible for storing and analyzing data. Both practical and logistical factors can be addressed by asking, Who? What? Where? When? Why? and How? For example:

1. Who will collect the data?

   - Examples: PT during the initial visit, office staff during initial paperwork

2. What kind of data/measurements will be collected?

   - Examples: Impairments, function, self-report questionnaires, global HRQOL questionnaires, disease-specific questionnaires

   - Are measurements reliable and valid?
   - What are the hallmarks of a "good" or "bad" outcome?

3. Where will data be collected?

4. When will data be collected?

   - Examples include: Initial visit, 4 weeks, after x number of visits, etc.

5. Why will you collect data?

   - How will the data be used? What is the purpose?
   - To whom will data be provided?

6. How will data be collected?

   - Procedures for ongoing data collection, tracking when data needs to be collected
   - Procedures for analysis and dissemination

Regardless of benefits that arise from good data collection and reporting, barriers exist.[2] Barriers include:

- Personnel resistance to incorporating ongoing consistent data collection procedures
- Differences in procedures for collecting data (variability in goniometric measurements or strength testing)
- Lack of appropriate, reliable, and valid tools to use
- Vast differences in patients with similar pathologies
- Time needed for storing, retrieving, analyzing, and reporting data.

A process must also be in place for consistent patient coding (ie, ICD-9), so that data retrieval is facilitated. In addition, organizations should consider direct and indirect costs such as the need for additional personnel or providing an employee time from normal duties to work with data or train staff. Another consideration is whether to use an outcomes management software package. These can be expensive to implement because of costs for hardware, software, upgrades, and report generation. Today, some outcomes measurement tools are being integrated into computerized documentation software such as APTA's Connect.

In summary, collecting outcomes data on groups of patients can be an arduous task, yet it has many benefits including providing justification of physical therapy services. Even if you choose not to collect or track data for research, understanding and identifying instruments' measurement properties can help to choose an instrument, facilitate goal writing, and document meaningful change in an individual patient's functional status.

# Review Questions

1. In your own words, define outcome.

2. Describe the PT's role in examining outcomes for individual patients.

3. Give an example of a patient cohort. Provide examples of outcomes data to be recorded in the discharge note that would be important for examining treatment effectiveness for these groups.

4. Compare and contrast generic (general health), disease-specific, and patient-specific instruments. Give positive and negative aspects of each.

5. Compare and contrast patient performance and patient self-report questionnaires. Give positive and negative aspects of each.

6. Define reliability and differentiate between intra-rater and inter-rater reliability.

7. How are reliability values reported?

8. What is the importance of knowing an instrument's SEM?

9. What types of validity are important when examining outcomes instruments?

10. What is responsiveness?

11. What statistics are often given when describing an instrument's responsiveness?

12. Which measurement property (besides reliability and validity) is most appropriate when determining which tool to use?

13. Which measurement property/properties help(s) you make decisions regarding change on individual patients?

# Application Exercises

1. Identify one functional outcome assessment tool and research its measurement properties. Describe the utility of the instrument in terms of reliability, validity, clinical utility, and responsiveness.

2. Identify one or two outcome measures for each of the following settings. Give their measurement properties (including reliability, validity, clinical utility, and responsiveness) and reference information when available. Determine if it is generic or disease-specific. Determine the administration technique (ie, patient performance or self-report).

a. Acute care setting

b. Inpatient rehabilitation unit

    i. Neurological disorder

    ii. Musculoskeletal disorder

c. Long-term care center

d. Skilled nursing unit

e. Home health

f. Outpatient Orthopedic clinic

    i. Upper extremity

    ii. Lower extremity

    iii. Spine

    iv. General

g. Cardiopulmonary patient (Dx: COPD) in home health

h. Pediatric Outpatient Clinic—Neurological Disorders

i. Pediatric Outpatient Clinic—Musculoskeletal Disorders

j. Pediatric-School setting—ages 5-9 years old

k. Early Intervention (Birth to three)

3. Identify a setting (like one listed in question 2) and a common diagnosis seen in that particular setting. Determine how you would go about implementing an outcomes assessment program for those patients.

4. Identify one clinician in your area and interview him or her regarding the use of outcomes assessment tools in the clinical setting. What instruments does he or she use? How are they used (ie, when is it administered, who administers it, how is it stored)? How has it influenced his or her practice? How has it influenced reimbursement? How is it incorporated into his or her documentation?

# References

1. American Physical Therapy Association. *The Guide to Physical Therapist Practice*. Alexandria, VA: APTA; 2001.

2. Ingersoll GL. Generating evidence through outcomes management. In: Melnyk BM, Fineout-Overholt E, eds. *Evidence-Based Practice in Nursing and Healthcare: A Guide to Best Practice*. Philadelphia, PA: Lippincott, Williams & Wilkins; 2005:299-332.

3. Hart DL. What should you expect from the study of clinical outcomes? (guest editorial). *J Orthop Sports Phys Ther*. 1998;28(1):1-2.

4. Finch E, Brooks D, Stratford PW, Mayo NE. *Physical Rehabilitation Outcomes Measures*. 2nd ed. Philadelphia, PA: Lippincott, Williams & Wilkins; 2002.

5. Westaway MD, Stratford PW, Binkley JM. The patient-specific functional scale. *J Orthop Sports Phys Ther*. 1998;27(5):331-8.

6. Portney LG, Watkins MP. *Foundations of Clinical Research: Applications to Practice*. 2nd ed. Upper Saddle River, NJ: Prentice Hall Health; 2000.

7. Domholdt E. *Physical Therapy Research: Principles and Applications*. 2nd ed. Philadelphia, PA: W.B. Saunders; 2000.

8. MacDermid JC, Stratford P. Applying evidence on outcome measures to hand therapy practice. *J Hand Ther*. 2004;17(2):165-73.

9. Michener LA, Leggin BG. A review of self-report scales for the assessment of hand function. *J Hand Ther*. 2001;14(2):68-76.

10. Beaton DE, Katz JN, Fossel AH, Wright JG, Tarasuk V. Measuring the whole or parts: validity, reliability, and responsiveness of the DASH outcome measure in different regions of the upper extremity. *J Hand Ther*. 2001;14(2):128-46.

11. Palombaro KM, Craik RL, Mangione KK, Tomlinson JD. Determining meaningful changes in gait speed after hip fracture. *Phys Ther*. 2006;86(6):809-16.

12. Lohr KN. Outcomes measurement: concepts and questions. *Inquiry*. 1988;25:37-50.

13. Jewell DV. Appraising evidence about outcomes. In: *Guide to Evidence-Based Physical Therapy*. Sudbury, MA: Jones and Bartlett Publishers; 2007:309-36.

14. Wakefield DS. Measuring health care outcomes: more work to do (guest editorial). *J Orthop Sports Phys Ther*. 1998;27(2):111-3.

## Chapter 11

# Legal, Regulatory, and Policy Issues in Documentation

*Ralph Utzman, PT, MPH, PhD*

## Chapter Objectives

Upon completion of this chapter, the reader will be able to:

1. Compare and contrast law, regulation, and policy.
2. Name at least two governmental agencies that develop regulations.
3. Describe the Health Insurance Portability and Accountability Act, including how it safeguards patient privacy.
4. Define malpractice, compliance, and informed consent.
5. Discuss how documentation can assist in managing risk of malpractice suits.
6. Describe the purpose of incident reports.
7. Identify how APTA's *Code of Ethics* and *Guide for Professional Conduct* relate to proper documentation.

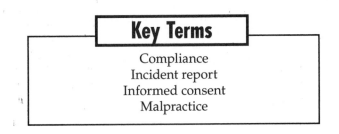

**Key Terms**

Compliance
Incident report
Informed consent
Malpractice

# Introduction

Physical therapists (PTs) and other health care professionals are heavily regulated. Patients are often placed in a vulnerable position due to illness or injury and rely on health care professionals who possess specialized knowledge and skills.[1] Often, public funds are used to pay for health care (see Chapter 12 for a detailed discussion of reimbursement issues). Laws, regulations, and organizational policies are written to protect patients from harm and to make sure that care is provided safely, effectively, and efficiently. The medical record is often used to document compliance with various laws, regulations, and policies. In cases where a patient sues a health care provider for negligence or malpractice, the medical record is often a key piece of evidence regarding how care was provided.

This chapter is not intended as a substitute for professional legal advice. Many health care facilities employ or retain licensed attorneys to assist with managing legal risks associated with providing health care. Other facilities, as well as therapists in private practice, can obtain legal advice from the insurance company from whom they purchase malpractice/liability coverage. Many organizations have "compliance officers" or departments that assist health care providers in understanding and following current regulations. Readers are urged to seek advice from one of these sources when confronted with specific questions in clinical practice.

# Law and Regulation

*Laws* are governmental statements of what we must do. They are developed by votes of Congress, state legislatures, or county/municipal governments. Laws can also result from court cases where a decision by a judge or jury sets a precedent for future cases. Laws often delegate oversight of a law to a government agency or regulatory body. This government agency may then write *regulations*, or rules that state how the intent of the law is to be carried out. Such regulations typically carry the force of law.[2]

## State Practice Acts and Licensure Boards

In all 50 states, laws exist that define what physical therapy is and who can practice physical therapy. These laws, which are enacted by state legislatures, are commonly known as *physical therapy practice acts*. In most states, these practice acts include provisions for a licensure board, which is a government agency that oversees practice of physical therapy. The licensure board, in turn, may write regulations that further describe parameters of practice. If a therapist fails to comply with either the practice act or regulations, the licensing board may suspend or revoke the therapist's license to practice.

For example, in West Virginia, the state legislature last modified the physical therapy practice act (WV Code Chapter 30, Article 20) in 2001. The practice act establishes that the WV Board of Physical Therapy is responsible for overseeing licensure of physical therapists in the state. The WV Board of Physical Therapy has published a series of regulations, entitled "Legislative Rules". One of these (Title 16, Series 1) provides definitions of the terms *physical therapist* and *physical therapist assistant* (PTA) that are somewhat more detailed than those in the statutory law. Series 1 also carefully defines how PTAs and other personnel are to be supervised in different care settings. These regulations have implications for documentation. Since a therapist's license can be suspended or revoked for violating regulations promulgated by the board (30-20-10.b.9) or for inappropriate utilization of support personnel (30-20-10.b.10), therapists in West Virginia should document appropriate direction and supervision of assistants in the medical record. All PTs should be familiar with the practice act and any associated regulations in the state(s) in which they are licensed.

# Medicare and Centers for Medicare & Medicaid Services

The previous chapter discussed general information about reimbursement and Medicare. Medicare is the largest payer for health care in the United States.[3] Medicare was created by Title XVIII of the Social Security Act in 1965 to provide health insurance coverage to older adults. Congress has passed several laws to modify the program over the years. For instance, legislation was passed in 1972 to include coverage for adults younger than 65 with certain long-term disabilities.[4] More recently, the Balanced Budget Act of 1998 modified the program by mandating implementation of cost control measures that had serious impact on the delivery of physical therapy services.[4]

The government agency responsible for oversight of the Medicare program is now known as the Center for Medicare and Medicaid Service (CMS). This agency maintains and regularly updates a large volume of regulations regarding payment for health care services provided to Medicare beneficiaries. One example is Chapter 15 of the *Medicare Benefits Policy Manual*. This regulation (as revised in June 2006) provides requirements for documentation of outpatient physical therapy services paid by Medicare Part B. Documentation-related provisions of the regulations include:

1. Documentation must demonstrate that services provided were reasonable, medically necessary, and skilled in nature.

2. The patient must be under the care of a physician, and the physical therapy plan of care must be certified by a physician every 30 days.

3. The physical therapy plan of care must include a diagnosis, long- and short-term goals, and

planned type, amount, duration, and frequency of treatment.

4. A progress report must be written by the PT every 30 days, or every 10 visits, whichever comes first.

5. A discharge report must be written at the conclusion of the patient's therapy episode.

The full text of the regulation can be downloaded from http://www.cms.hhs.gov/Transmittals/downloads/R52BP.pdf

## Health Insurance Portability and Accountability Act of 1996 (HIPAA)

Another example of a federal law that impacts PTs is the Health Insurance Portability and Accountability Act (HIPAA). Title I of HIPAA allows workers to maintain their insurance coverage when they change jobs. Title II focuses on preventing fraud and abuse, and required the US Department of Health and Human Services (DHHS) to establish rules for safeguarding the privacy of a patient's personal health information.[5]

The final privacy rule developed by DHHS went into effect on April 14, 2003. Health care providers, health insurance plans, and health information clearinghouses are subject to the rule if they hold or transmit protected health information in any form —oral, written, facsimile, or electronic. Protected health information includes all personal health information, including medical records and other identifiable health information.[5] Electronic media refers to the Internet, intranets and extranets, leased lines, dial up lines, private networks, or transmissions occurring through magnetic tape, disk, or compact disk.[6] Under the privacy rule, patients are granted several rights, including those listed below.

- The right to read and get copies of their own medical records.

- The right to make amendments to their own medical records.

- The right to know who has access to their medical records.

- The right to give written permission prior to disclosure of their personal health information.

- The right to file a complaint when they believe their privacy is not being protected.[7]

The privacy rule allows health care providers to share information without written consent in circumstances that relate to routine care of the patient. Such circumstances would include providing information to a physician or other health care provider involved in the patient's care, or providing copies of medical records to insurance companies for reimbursement purposes. Such disclosures should only provide the minimum information necessary to accomplish the purpose.[6]

Under the HIPAA privacy rule, health care providers must obtain consent prior to releasing patients' protected health information for other reasons, such as marketing or research.[7] For instance, if a PT or student is writing a case study on a patient, the author must obtain patient consent first. However, the material may be used without consent if it is first "de-identified." This means that any information that could potentially be used to identify the patient must be removed. The rule lists 18 elements that must be removed (Table 11-1); in addition the author would need to be sure that the patient could not be identified in any way from the remaining information.[8] These elements may be removed electronically or manually. Research protocols must be designed in ways that safeguard patient privacy, and these methods must be approved by an Institutional Review Board.[8]

The privacy rule requires health care facilities to provide training related to patient privacy safeguards to their employees. Facilities are also required to designate a privacy officer to oversee employee training and overall implementation of privacy safeguards.[5] Many states have laws regarding privacy of personal health information. If the state law is more stringent than the HIPAA privacy rule, the state law supersedes HIPAA.[7]

# Legal Issues

## Malpractice and Risk Management

Good documentation is the cornerstone of good risk management (Table 11-2). Anytime a PT provides care to a patient, the therapist is taking a legal risk.[9] Malpractice lawsuits can result from professional negligence, intentional misconduct by the health care provider, injury resulting from the use of defective equipment, or poor outcomes related to the use of high-risk procedures.[10] Many facilities employ risk managers, or utilize risk management committees or departments, whose responsibilities include minimizing potential risks for health care providers involved with patient/client management. These individuals or groups investigate complaints or concerns as they are brought forth, either by patients or providers. An important aspect of their investigation is examining the medical record and other available documentation. The documentation allows the risk manager(s) to "determine if the care provided met the standard of care required of prudent health care providers."[9]

Price[9] identified two important risk management documents. First, *informed consent* documents provide evidence of the patient's agreement to or rejection of a recommended treatment after being provided with

---

Table 11-1

# Data to Be Removed to "De-Identify" Patient Records

- Names
- All elements of address smaller than the state
- All elements of dates related to the patient (such as birthdate), except the year.
- Phone numbers
- Facsimile numbers
- Electronic mail addresses
- Social security number
- Medical record numbers
- Insurance numbers
- Account numbers
- Certificate/license numbers
- Vehicle identification, registration, and license plate numbers
- Identifiers (serial numbers) of medical devices
- Internet addresses (URLs)
- Internet protocol (IP) address numbers
- Fingerprints, voice prints, and other biometric data
- Full-face photographs or similar images that could be used to identify the patient
- Any other unique identifier, code, or characteristic

Source: National Institutes of Health. Protecting Personal Health Information in Research: Understanding the HIPAA Privacy Rule [NIH website]. April 14, 2003. Available at: http://privacyruleandresearch.nih.gov/pr_02.asp. Accessed September 17, 2007.

---

Table 11-2

# Tips for Documentation and Risk Management

- Document at the time care is provided, or at the soonest available opportunity. The longer you wait, the more likely you will forget important details.
- Stay abreast of APTA documentation guidelines, billing and coding procedures, and policies and procedures of your institution, and follow them.
- Make sure that documentation demonstrates your decision-making process.[9,15]
- Document informed consent.[10]
- Document instructions to patients.[15]
- Document patient compliance/adherence. Lewis[15] suggests careful documentation of patient appointment cancellations. It is also important to include notations regarding whether the patient followed his/her home exercise program and safety precautions.
- Do not include copies of incident reports in the medical record, or mention them in the patient's chart.[10,14] Document the incident and the care provided in the patient's record as objectively as possible, then forward the (separate) incident report to your institution's risk manager.

a clear, thorough explanation of its risks, benefits, and available alternatives. The patient must also be provided with information on the probability of success of the treatment as well as the consequences of having no treatment at all.[9,11,12] The PT is responsible for obtaining informed consent prior to providing any intervention.[1]

Suppose that a therapist performs a stretching technique on a patient following tendon repair surgery. Even though an appropriate amount of time has elapsed since the surgery and the patient's surgeon has verified that gentle stretching may begin, there is still a chance that even gentle stretching may cause the repaired tendon to rupture. The therapist explains this, along with other treatment alternatives, to the patient before beginning the treatment session. The patient gives consent, and the therapist proceeds with stretching. After a few treatment sessions, the tendon is re-ruptured. Hopefully, the therapist documented discussing the risks and alternatives to stretching, as well as the patient's consent. If the therapist did not, and the patient sued for malpractice, no proof would exist that informed consent was obtained.

Another important document is the *incident report*. Incident reports are used to document "errors and departures from expected procedures or outcomes."[13] A report prepared by the University of California at San Francisco outlined three categories of critical incidents that should be recorded: adverse outcomes to a treatment that has been provided, procedural breakdowns, and catastrophic events.[13] Examples in physical therapy include patients falling during gait training, accidental burns from hot packs or other modalities, confidentiality breaches, or any other event that may cause harm to a patient or visitor within or around the facility. Incident reports can serve as a basis for improving care by identifying and investigating problems as they arise.[9] Incident reports also provide an internal account in case legal action results from the adverse event.[10] Incident reports should be filed with risk management departments, and not included in the patient's medical record.[10,14]

## Fraud and Abuse

Each year, Medicare and its beneficiaries pay millions of dollars toward fraudulent claims.[16] Insurance fraud can be defined as billing a third-party payer for services that were never provided or billing for an item or service that is reimbursed at a higher rate than the service that was actually provided.[17] Fraud is a crime and is punishable by law. The US DHHS, the Office of the Inspector General, the Federal Bureau of Investigation, and the Department of Justice all take part in preventing and detecting Medicare fraud.[16]

Another improper billing procedure is abuse. Abuse occurs when a provider bills for items that are not covered or misuses billing codes.[17] Abuse differs from fraud in that fraud is intentional, while abuse often results from unintended billing errors or poor awareness of proper billing and coding procedures.

In order to avoid accusations of abuse, PTs should stay abreast of current reimbursement and coding guidelines. Accurate billing with corresponding documentation can help prevent fraud accusations.

Insurance fraud and abuse are both illegal and unethical. The APTA *Guide for Professional Conduct*[1] states that physical therapists "shall not make statements that he/she knows or should know are false, deceptive, fraudulent or unfair." Principle 7 of the APTA *Code of Ethics*[18] states that PTs shall only seek payments that are deserved and reasonable.

# Organizational Policies

While laws and regulations are written by the government and its agencies, *policies* are rules written by non-governmental organizations. Such organizations include professional associations (eg, APTA) or accrediting bodies (eg, Joint Commission on Accreditation of Health Care Organizations, or JCAHO). Health care organizations, like hospitals and clinics, also develop policies that govern their employees. A primary purpose of organizational policy is to standardize the actions and behaviors of members of that organization. Organizational policies can also serve to communicate the values and philosophies that guide members' behaviors.

This text has already introduced readers to several APTA policies that relate directly to documentation. The APTA *Code of Ethics*[18] and *Guide for Professional Conduct*[1] both support the importance of proper documentation (Principles 2, 3, and 7). *The Guide for Physical Therapist Practice*,[19] and the Patient/Client Management Model on which it is based, serve as a foundation for clinical decision making. Documentation should flow from and demonstrate the clinical decision-making process. This is reflected in the APTA's *Guidelines for Physical Therapy Documentation*.[20] Together, these documents establish the standard of practice for documenting physical therapy care.

Individual health care organizations should have policies that describe how exactly PTs within the institution should document. Ideally, these institutional policies should be based on the standard of practice outlined by the APTA. They may also be influenced by accreditation standards and requirements of third-party payers. Well-written policies will take into account the information technologies used within the facility (ie, paper-based vs. electronic medical records); the mechanisms for storage, retrieval, and transmission; safeguards for patient privacy; and best practices for managing legal risks.

By becoming a member (or an employee) of an organization, the member either implicitly or explicitly agrees to follow the policies of that organization. Failure to follow those policies may result in penalties such as suspension or dismissal. Organizational policies can also be indirectly binding on nonmembers if those policies represent an accepted standard of practice. For instance, say a PT chooses not to be a member of the APTA. The therapist and a PTA are working with an elderly patient who recently had surgical repair of a fractured femur. During the course of treatment, the femur is re-fractured, requiring further surgery. The patient and her family file a malpractice lawsuit, claiming that the therapist and assistant were both negligent in providing care. Even though the therapist is not a member of the APTA, attorneys for both the patient and the therapist will likely compare the medical record to APTA's documentation guidelines. Adherence to these guidelines will be presented to the jury, who will ultimately decide whether the standard of care was met, and whether the therapist and assistant are liable for the patient's re-injury.

---

# Review Questions

1.  What are the differences between statutory and case law?

2.  What are the differences between law and regulation? What are the similarities?

3.  What functions do state boards of physical therapy (state licensing boards) serve?

4.  What is CMS, and what does it do?

5.  What are the purposes of HIPAA? What rights does it give to patients? What requirements does it place on health care providers and organizations for protecting patient privacy?

6.  Compare and contrast *fraud* and *abuse*.

7.  Describe documentation strategies for managing malpractice risks.

8.  What types of occurrences should be documented on incident reports? How and where should incident reports be filed?

9.  What is an organizational policy? How is a policy binding on members of the organization? How might an organizational policy affect individuals who are not members of the organization?

# Application Exercises

1. Obtain copies of the physical therapy practice act (statutory law) and rules/regulations for your state. Review the documents and answer the following:

   a. What is the scope of practice of a PT? A PTA? Are there any limitations regarding what a PTA is allowed to document, compared to a PT?

   b. What are the rules for supervision of PTAs and other support personnel?

   c. Is a referral required for a patient to receive physical therapy services? If so, who may refer? If there are provisions for direct access (evaluation and/or treatment without referral), are there any limitations or restrictions?

   d. What rules apply to authenticating (signing) entries in the medical record? What initials should follow the PTs name? If the PT has a DPT degree, may he/she use this designation? Is the PT required to include his/her license number?

   e. What are the potential consequences for practice inconsistent with the practice act and/or rules? How are disciplinary procedures carried out?

2. Obtain copies of the practice act and rules/regulations for another state. Or, obtain a copy of the Model Practice Act developed by the Federation of State Boards of Physical Therapy. Compare and contrast the document with the document you reviewed in Exercise 1.

3. Review your organization's policies and procedures for HIPAA compliance.

# References

1. American Physical Therapy Association Ethics and Judicial Committee. Guide for Professional Conduct. Available at: http://www.apta.org/AM/Template.cfm?Section=Home&Template=/CM/HTMLDisplay.cfm&ContentID=24781. Accessed December 30, 2006.

2. Wing KR. *Law and the Public's Health*. 4th ed. Ann Arbor, MI: Health Administration Press; 1995.

3. Sandstrom RW, Lohman H, Bramble JD. *Health Services: Policy and Systems for Therapists*. Upper Saddle River, NJ: Prentice Hall; 2003.

4. American Physical Therapy Association. *The Reimbursement Resource Book*. Alexandria, VA: 2005.

5. Nosse LJ, Friberg DG, Kovacek PR. *Managerial and Supervisory Principles for Phyiscal Therapists*. 2nd ed. Philadelphia, PA: Lippincott, Williams & Wilkins; 2005:52-65.

6. Ravitz KS. The HIPAA privacy final modified rule. *PT—Magazine of Physical Therapy*. 2002;10(11)21-25.

7. Office of Civil Rights. HIPAA Fact Sheet. Available at: http://www.hhs.gov/news/facts/privacy.html. Accessed June 1, 2004.

8. National Institutes of Health. Protecting Personal Health Information in Research: Understanding the HIPAA Privacy Rule [NIH website]. April 14, 2003. Available at: http://privacyrule-andresearch.nih.gov/pr_02.asp. Accessed September 17, 2007.

9. Price SA. Risk Management. Presented at West Virginia Physical Therapy Association Chapter Meeting. Aug 9 1997; Flatwoods, WV.

10. Scott R. *Legal Aspects of Documenting Patient Care*. Gaithersburg, MD: Aspen Publishers; 2000.

11. Boyle RJ. Process of informed consent. In: Fletcher JC, Lombardo PA, Marshall MF, Miller FG, eds. *Introduction to Clinical Ethics*. 2nd ed. Hagerstown, MD: University Publishing Group; 1997:89-105.

12. Smith LC. Risk management: the hot topics. *PT—Magazine of Physical Therapy*. 2000;8(12):26-33.

13. Agency for Healthcare Research and Quality. Making health care safer: a critical analysis of patient safety practices. Evidence Report/Technology Assessment: No. 43. AHRQ Publication No.01-E058. Available at: http://www.ahrq.gov/clinic/ptsafety/ . Accessed December 15, 2007.

14. Nosse LJ, Friberg DG, Kovacek PR. *Managerial and Supervisory Principles for Physical Therapists*. 2nd ed. Philadelphia, PA: Lippincott, Williams & Wilkins; 2005:458-79.

15. Lewis DK. Do the write thing: document everything. *PT—Magazine of Physical Therapy*. 2002;10(7):30-34.

16. Centers for Medicare and Medicaid Services. Fraud Overview. Available at: http://www.medicare.gov/FraudAbuse/Overview.asp. Accessed December 15, 2007.

17. Centers for Medicare and Medicaid Services. Medicare Glossary. Available at: http://www.medicare.gov/Glossary/Search.asp. Accessed December 15, 2007.

18. American Physical Therapy Association. *Code of Ethics* (HOD S06-00-12-23). Available at: http://www.apta.org/AM/Template.cfm?Section=Home&Template=/CM/HTMLDisplay.cfm&ContentID=25854. Accessed December 15, 2007.

19. American Physical Therapy Association. *The Guide to Physical Therapist Practice*. Alexandria, VA: APTA; 2001.

20. American Physical Therapy Association. *Guidelines: Physical Therapy Documentation of Patient/Client Management*. Alexandria, VA; 2006. Report No. BOD G03-05-16-41.

## Chapter 12

# Documentation and Reimbursement

*Ralph Utzman, PT, MPH, PhD*

## Chapter Objectives

Upon completion of this chapter, the reader will be able to:

1. Define the terms third-party payment, premium, deductible, copayment, prospective payment, fee for service.
2. Describe who pays for health care in the United States.
3. Describe the processes used for third-party reimbursement.
4. Describe how clinical documentation is linked with reimbursement.
5. Describe documentation strategies that help maximize reimbursement.

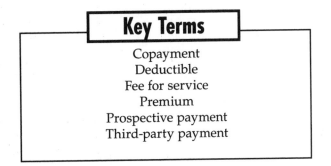

### Key Terms

Copayment
Deductible
Fee for service
Premium
Prospective payment
Third-party payment

# Introduction

Traditionally, information about billing and reimbursement has been kept separate from the medical record. As noted in Chapter 2, documentation has gradually become more intertwined with the process of receiving payment for health care services. This chapter will introduce the reader to key reimbursement concepts and illustrate how insurance companies and other payers use our documentation to make reimbursement decisions. Finally, the chapter will provide practical suggestions to help therapists avoid payment denials. Throughout the chapter, the term *payer* will be used to refer to third parties (such as insurance companies) who pay for health care services. The term *provider* will be used to refer to those who provide health care, such as physical therapists (PTs), physicians, and hospitals.

# Who Pays for Health Care?

When you go to the mall and buy a pair of shoes, there are generally two parties involved in the transaction. The first party is the customer, who selects and pays for the shoes. The second party is the store itself, which provides the shoes in exchange for payment. In contrast, payment for health care usually involves a third party—an insurance company, for example—who pays for the services provided to the patient. Sometimes, the patient will pay the bill and then receive reimbursement from an insurance company. More typically, health care providers are paid directly by the third-party payer.

Third-party payers can be categorized in several ways. First, some are public and some are private. Many people have private insurance, an arrangement in which an insurance company receives a monthly payment, or premium, for every person who is enrolled in the insurance plan. In some cases, individuals pay this monthly premium themselves. More commonly, the individual's employer pays the premium (either partially or entirely) as a benefit of employment. The insurance company pools these premiums and uses them to pay for the health care costs of all those who are enrolled in the insurance program. Other people are covered by public insurance programs run by the government. These public plans use money collected through tax payments, rather than monthly premiums, to pay for health care. Common public plans include Medicare, which is the federal program that pays for health care for older adults and people with certain disabilities. Another common public payer is Medicaid. This program is paid for through a combination of state and federal tax dollars, and covers health care costs for those with low incomes.

In 2006, 53% of Americans had employer-based insurance, while 25% had public coverage (ie, Medicare or Medicaid).[1] Six percent either paid for their own insurance premiums, or they had coverage through other public programs.[1] An increasing number of Americans (16% in 2005[1]) are uninsured, meaning that they do not have access to third-party payment and must pay out-of-pocket for all the health care services they receive.

# Cost Containment and Managed Care

The costs of health care in the United States have been rising since the 1950s. The increases in costs are in part due to improvements in technology, advances in clinical practice, and specialization of health care providers. However, the increased costs can also be attributed to the incentives provided by our third-party payment system.[2,3] Consider the earlier example of buying a pair of shoes. If you have a limited amount of money, you might shop around at several stores to check prices. You end up at a discount store and buy shoes that are on sale because they are leftovers from last year. However, if a faceless stranger offers to pay for your shoes, you may decide to buy shoes of the newest style from a trendy boutique, regardless of the price. And the boutique, knowing that the faceless stranger will pay whatever price is charged, has no incentive to offer discounted prices and every incentive to sell as many shoes as possible.

Even though shoes and health care are very different products, you can see how insurance coverage may affect the priorities of both patients and providers. Patients understandably want the best care possible. Providers want to provide that care. Costs rise, in part, because patients are not responsible for paying the full price of the care they receive.[3] These costs are passed on to the insurance program.

The problem is that the third-party payers have to come up with the money to pay for increasingly larger health care bills. This increases the cost of doing business for employers who pay for their workers' insurance premiums. The increased costs of Medicare and Medicaid lead to increased taxes for everyone. Not surprisingly, payers have developed mechanisms to control costs.

One common strategy for containing costs is to make the patient responsible for paying part of the bill through deductibles and copayments. For instance, a patient with a $500 deductible would pay for the first $500 worth of care he receives each year, and then the insurance would pay for the rest.[4] A patient with a $10 copayment must pay $10 for each instance of service provided (doctor visit, prescription refill, therapy session), with the insurance covering the remaining charge for each service.[4] Payers also use a variety of methods to control provider behavior. For instance, providers may be required to request authorization from the insurance company before providing treatment. Some services, like physical therapy, may need to be reauthorized after a certain amount of time or visits. Over the past 20 years, the use of cost containment strategies has increased to the point where insurance companies actually manage the care patients receive. Managed care plans restrict patients' choice of providers and use a variety of strategies to control costs, while streamlining processes to provide for more efficient care.[5]

# Processes for Third-Party Reimbursement

Why is it important to know about health care costs and cost containment? Most PTs want to provide the best possible care for their patients. In order for therapists to be paid for their services, we need to understand how we are paid for our services and what documentation is required. The process of requesting payment from a third-party payer is called *submitting a claim*. Depending on the payer and the care setting, the mechanisms for payment and claims filing vary.

## Fee for Service

*Fee for service* is the oldest method of payment and is still used by many payers today. A common example in physical therapy is Medicare Part B. Medicare Part B pays for physician fees and various other outpatient services, such as physical therapy, for older adults.[3] The health care provider is paid a fee for each service or procedure provided to a patient. Although the provider sets prices for each procedure or service, it is more common for the provider to be paid based on a predetermined fee schedule. In some cases (eg, Medicare), the fee schedule is determined by the payer and updated on a regular basis.[3] In other cases, the provider may negotiate with the payer to set the fee schedule.

To submit a claim, the provider documents the patient's diagnosis and the services provided on a claim form. Diagnoses are coded using ICD-9 codes (*International Classification of Diseases, Ninth Edition*). This coding system categorizes illnesses and injuries by cause and body system.[5] Each diagnosis is coded as a three digit number, and can contain an additional two digits to help specify disease characteristics and locations.

Procedures and services are coded using CPT (Common Procedural Terminology) codes.[5] The American Medical Association develops and maintains the extensive listing of CPT codes, which represent a broad range of health care services and procedures provided by physicians and other health care providers.

After care is provided to the patient, the appropriate ICD-9 and CPT codes are documented on a claim form, which the provider submits (either in paper form or electronically) to the payer. Before paying for the services, the payer usually reviews the bill to make sure that the services provided (and coded by CPT codes) were appropriate given the patient's diagnosis (as coded by ICD-9 codes). If questions arise, the payer may request a copy of the patient's record. There are several reasons that a payer may deny payment for a claim. Some common reasons are:

- The claim form was incomplete or not filled in correctly.
- Documentation was illegible.[6]
- The care documented in the medical record did not match the care billed on the claim form.
- The documentation does not demonstrate that skilled care was provided (see Chapter 2).[6]
- The documentation does not demonstrate that the care provided was reasonable and/or medically necessary (see Chapter 2).[6]
- The documentation did not include proof of referral from a physician. Many insurers require patients to have a referral from their doctor before they will pay for physical therapy. Medicare Part B requires that a physician approve of the PT's plan of care every 30 days.[7]

In addition, payers may place limits on the amount of care provided. For example, Medicare Part B currently caps the amount of outpatient physical therapy a person can receive per year (currently $1,740 per calendar year as of this writing).[6] Other payers may limit the number of visits a patient can receive. It is important for providers to know these restrictions as well as how to appeal or request extensions for care in case a patient needs care beyond the limits. In all cases, careful, accurate documentation is vital for providing the best care possible for the patient and receiving payment for services provided.

## Prospective Payment Systems

Fee for service payment as described above can encourage over-utilization of services, since each service or procedure provided at every visit is paid separately. In order to rein in costs, payers have developed *prospective payment systems* (PPS) that pay the provider a set amount of money instead of paying for each item separately.[3] The federal government developed the first Medicare PPS in 1983 to slow growth in hospital costs.[8] In the late 1990s, other PPS systems were developed for skilled nursing, home health, and inpatient rehabilitation.

### Acute Care

Medicare Part A pays for hospitalization for older adults. Prior to 1983, Medicare paid hospitals using a fee schedule that was based on the hospital's costs. In 1983, a PPS was introduced which radically changed how hospitals are paid. Hospitals are now paid a set fee based on the patient's diagnosis.[8]

For example, suppose a 72-year-old woman is admitted to the hospital for surgery to repair a humerus fracture. Under the old system, Medicare would have received a bill in which every procedure and service provided to the patient would be billed separately. Every medication, every bandage change, and every PT session would be billed as a separate line item. Under the current PPS system, the hospital is paid a lump sum to cover the patient's entire hospital stay. This lump sum covers all the care provided to the patient.

So how does Medicare decide how much to pay the hospital? Upon discharge, the hospital assigns an ICD-9 code to the patient that describes her primary diagnosis at discharge. Medicare uses *Diagnosis Related Groups* (DRGs), which is a fee schedule based on groups of ICD-9 codes, to determine how much to pay the hospital.[3] The DRG system encourages the hospital to provide efficient and effective care. If the patient gets well and is able to return home quickly, the hospital gets to keep any money left over. However, if the patient does not improve quickly and stays in the hospital too long, the hospital loses money.

In order for acute care hospitals to stay in business under the DRG system, care must be provided efficiently. For PTs who practice in these facilities, communication and coordination with other health care providers is vital. The patient's functional status, the physical therapy plan of care, the interventions performed, and the patient's response to those interventions must all be carefully documented.

## Skilled Nursing Facilities

In 1997, Congress enacted the Balanced Budget Act. This law included provisions for reducing Medicare costs.[3] The law charged Medicare with the task of implementing PPS systems in other areas of care besides acute care hospitals. The first of these PPS systems to be implemented under the act was in Skilled Nursing Facilities (SNF).

SNFs provide continuing care to patients who are no longer in need of acute care hospitalization but still require skilled nursing or rehabilitative services that cannot be provided in the patient's home. Documentation must show that skilled care was provided and that the care was reasonable and medically necessary. If these conditions are met, Medicare will pay for up to 100 days per year of skilled care.[9]

Medicare pays the SNF a daily rate based on patient acuity. To determine patient acuity, the patient is evaluated by nurses and therapists using a standardized tool called the *Minimum Data Set* (MDS), Version 2.0. The MDS records how much assistance the patient needs as well as the number of minutes of skilled care the patient receives. After the MDS is completed, the patient is categorized into a *Resource Utilization Group* (RUG) that determines the daily rate that the SNF will be paid.[5] The MDS tool and instructions for use are available at: http://www.cms.hhs.gov/NursingHome QualityInits/20_NHQIMDS20.asp.

### Home Health Care

The Balanced Budget Act also brought changes in how Medicare pays home health agencies. Similar to SNFs, home health agencies are now paid based on an interdisciplinary evaluation of patient acuity. The tool used in home health agencies is called the *Outcome and Assessment Information Set* (OASIS). Based on this evaluation, the home health agency is paid a fixed amount for a 60-day episode of care.[5,10] The home health agency must use that money as efficiently as possible by providing the appropriate amount of care at the right time.

The OASIS tool is available for download from the CMS website at: http://www.cms.hhs.gov/HomeHeal thQualityInits/12_HHQIOASISDataSet.asp.

### Inpatient Rehabilitation

The final setting affected by the Balanced Budget Act was inpatient rehabilitation. Similar to home health and SNF settings, the staff performs an interdisciplinary evaluation of the patient, which is documented on a standardized tool called the *Patient Assessment Instrument* (PAI).[11] The PAI includes a functional assessment called Functional Independence Measure (FIM). The patient's FIM score, diagnosis, and comorbidities are used to classify the patient into a *Case Mix Group* (CMG). The rehabilitation facility is then paid a fixed amount, based on the patient's CMG classification, to pay for the patient's entire stay.[11] The PAI tool is available for download from the CMS website at: http://www.cms.hhs.gov/InpatientRehabFacPPS/ downloads/CMS-10036.pdf

Under all prospective payment systems, complete and accurate documentation is vital to effective, efficient care and adequate reimbursement. The medical record is the primary tool for communication between members of the health care team. PTs must be skilled at accurately assessing and documenting each patient's functional status and developing an efficient, effective plan of care. PTs are responsible for managing and documenting the implementation of the plan of care and the patient's progress.

# Documentation Strategies to Avoid Payment Denials

This book provides a foundation for documenting physical therapy care that is consistent with professional standards of practice. The good news is that documenting according to the standards of practice is helpful in maximizing reimbursement. Following are some points to keep in mind.

## Make Sure Documentation and Billing Are Accurate and Consistent

Never assume that you are the only one who will see the patient's medical record. It is not uncommon for payers to request copies of your documentation to review. Your documentation must be complete and support the treatment that was provided.[5] This includes documenting the time spent providing skilled care. Many CPT codes are time-based. For example, 97110 is the CPT code representing therapeutic exercise to improve range of motion, strength, and endurance.[5] It specifies that 15 minutes of exercise should be performed when using this code. Therefore, the provider should carefully document the time involved in providing the intervention to justify reimbursement.

## Always Write Legibly

Illegible documentation is as bad as no documentation. If claims reviewers can't read your writing, the reimbursement claim will be denied.

## Document Medical Necessity

Chapter 2 discusses the concept of medical necessity. Keep in mind that an accurate diagnosis is needed, but not sufficient on its own, to demonstrate medical necessity. When documenting the patient's history, you must document how and when the patient's functional status changed.

Besides documentation of the patient's history, you should choose reliable, valid tests and measurements that will allow you to objectively document the patient's functional status and impairments.[5] (Please refer to Chapter 10 for more information on documenting outcomes.) It is recommended that you choose numeric measures (the 0/5 to 5/5 scale for manual muscle testing, for example) rather than categorical descriptions (normal, good, fair, poor, trace, none) when appropriate, because numeric measures are more easily understood. You should use the best functional outcome measures available for your patient. This may require that you research various tools and their validity, reliability, and sensitivity. Besides making a case for medical necessity, the right measure can be helpful in demonstrating progress over time.

Finally, your documentation must demonstrate how your plan of care will alleviate the patient's impairments and functional limitations. The initial note should demonstrate your problem-solving process, and interim notes should show progress over time.

## Document Skill

In order to be reimbursed, your documentation must reflect that the skills of a PT are needed and that ongoing care is provided by skilled personnel. For example, compare these two statements from a patient plan of care:

"The patient will ambulate with assistance twice daily."

"Gait training twice daily, emphasizing proper weight bearing and moderate assistance for balance and sequencing, progressing from the parallel bars to a walker as patient gait improves."

From the first statement, the reader might infer that anyone could walk with the patient and that skilled care is not necessary. The second statement, however, makes it clear that skilled care is necessary for safety, assistance, instruction, and progression.

## Avoid Repetitive Charting and Ban Throwaway Words

The life of a PT is hectic, and it's very easy to fall into repetitive charting habits. While efficiency is important, you should never trade time for quality. Repetitive charting habits can lead to documentation that doesn't demonstrate skill, problem solving, or patient progress.

For example, you should never use the term "Tolerated treatment well" as your assessment in a daily note.[11] Statements like these provide no information on how the patient actually tolerated the treatment. Was the patient less tired? Was the patient pain-free? Could the patient perform his or her home program? Did the patient have questions, and how were these questions addressed? Similarly, avoid statements like "Cont. as above" either as your intervention or your care plan. These types of phrases don't show that the patient has progressed, or that treatment has been adjusted accordingly.

## Review Questions

1. What is a third-party payer?

2. What is the difference between a premium and a copayment? How might these mechanisms influence patient behavior with respect to seeking health care?

3. What is managed care?

4. How does fee for service payment work?

5. What is prospective payment?

6. How does Medicare reimburse for care provided in acute care hospitals? Rehabilitation hospitals/units? Skilled nursing facilities? Home health?

7. What are ICD-9 codes and CPT codes used for?

8. What documentation habits can help you maximize reimbursement for your services?

## Application Exercises

1. Review the interim notes you wrote for Application Exercise 5 in Chapter 9. Using the strategies for avoiding claims denials listed on p. 167, critique the notes.

2. Review an initial examination and interim notes written by a classmate or colleague. Critique the notes from a payer's viewpoint.

3. Obtain copies of the Inpatient Rehabilitation PAI and Home Health OASIS forms used by Medicare (internet links for these appear in this chapter). Compare and contrast these two forms. What part(s) of the forms would a PT complete? How much time would it take to complete the documentation? How might accuracy affect reimbursement?

4. In the clinic, choose a patient and follow the patient's reimbursement claim from filing to final payment. During the process, take note of how many people had access to the patient's medical record. Was payment obtained on the first attempt? If not, how could the documentation be improved to prevent future denials?

# References

1. Kaiser Family Foundation. State Health Facts. Available at: URL: http://www.statehealthfacts.org/cgi-bin/healthfacts.cgi?action=compare&category=Health+Coverage+%26+Uninsured&subcategory=Health+Insurance+Status&topic=Total+Population. Accessed December 21, 2006.

2. Rasmussen B. *Reimbursement and Fiscal Management in Rehabilitation*. Alexandria, VA: American Physical Therapy Association; 1995.

3. Sandstrom RW, Lohman H, Bramble JD. *Health Services: Policy and Systems for Therapists*. Upper Saddle River, NJ: Prentice Hall; 2003.

4. Nosse LJ, Friberg DG, Kovacek PR. *Managerial and Supervisory Principles for Physical Therapists*. 2nd ed. Philadelphia, PA: Lippincott, Williams & Wilkins; 2005:21-38.

5. American Physical Therapy Association. *The Reimbursement Resource Book*. Alexandria, VA: 2005.

6. Centers for Medicare and Medicaid Services. Medicare Benefit Policy Manual: Chapter 15 – Covered Medical and Other Health Services. Transmittal 52; June 30, 2006.

7. Palmetto GBA. Medicare Part B: Physical Therapy Services. September 2006. Available at: http://www.palmettogba.com/palmetto/providers.nsf/Attachments/0F3D3B5D8B1E55A98525725F00448DD0/$FILE/Therapy+Services.pdf. Accessed September 4, 2007.

8. Cleverly WO. Financial environment. In: *Essentials of Health Care Finance*. 4th ed. Gaithersburg, MD: Aspen Publishers; 1997:10-24.

9. Centers for Medicare and Medicaid Services. Medicare and You 2007. Washington, DC: US Department of Health and Human Services. July 1, 2007. Available at: http://www.medicare.gov/Publications/Pubs/pdf/10050.pdf. Accessed September 4, 2007.

10. Centers for Medicare and Medicaid Services. Home Health PPS Overview [CMS website]. December 7, 2006. Available at: http://www.cms.hhs.gov/HomeHealthPPS/01_overview.asp. Accessed September 4, 2007.

11. Centers for Medicare and Medicaid Services. Inpatient Rehabilitation Facility PPS Overview [CMS website]. October 27, 2006. Available at: http://www.cms.hhs.gov/InpatientRehabFacPPS/. Accessed September 4, 2007.

12. Clifton DW. "Tolerated treatment well" may no longer be tolerated. *PT—Magazine of Physical Therapy*. 1995;3(10):24.

# Appendices

# Appendix A: APTA Guidelines for Physical Therapy Documentation of Patient/Client Management

BOD G03-05-16-41 (Program 32) [Amended BOD 02-02-16-20; BOD 11-01-06-10; BOD 03-01-16-51; BOD 03-00-22-54; BOD 03-99-14-41; BOD 11-98-19-69; BOD 03-97-27-69; BOD 03-95-23-61; BOD 11-94-33-107; BOD 06-93-09-13; Initial BOD 03-93-21-55] [Guideline]

## Preamble

The American Physical Therapy Association (APTA) is committed to meeting the physical therapy needs of society, to meeting the needs and interests of its members, and to developing and improving the art and science of physical therapy, including practice, education and research. To help meet these responsibilities, the APTA Board of Directors has approved the following guidelines for physical therapy documentation. It is recognized that these guidelines do not reflect all of the unique documentation requirements associated with the many specialty areas within the physical therapy profession. Applicable for both hand written and electronic documentation systems, these guidelines are intended to be used as a foundation for the development of more specific documentation guidelines in clinical areas, while at the same time providing guidance for the physical therapy profession across all practice settings. Documentation may also need to address additional regulatory or payer requirements.

Finally, be aware that these guidelines are intended to address documentation of patient/client management, not to describe the provision of physical therapy services. Other APTA documents, including APTA *Standards of Practice for Physical Therapy, Code of Ethics* and *Guide for Professional Conduct*, and *The Guide to Physical Therapist Practice*, address provision of physical therapy services and patient/client management.

## APTA Position on Documentation

### *Documentation Authority For Physical Therapy Services*

Physical therapy examination, evaluation, diagnosis, prognosis, and intervention shall be documented, dated, and authenticated by the physical therapist who performs the service. Intervention provided by the physical therapist or selected interventions provided by the physical therapist assistant is documented, dated, and authenticated by the physical therapist or, when permissible by law, the physical therapist assistant.

Other notations or flow charts are considered a component of the documented record but do not meet the requirements of documentation in or of themselves.

Students in physical therapist or physical therapist assistant programs may document when the record is additionally authenticated by the physical therapist or, when permissible by law, documentation by physical therapist assistant students may be authenticated by a physical therapist assistant.

## Operational Definitions

### *Guidelines*

APTA defines a "guideline" as a statement of advice.

### *Authentication*

The process used to verify that an entry is complete, accurate and final. Indications of authentication can include original written signatures and computer "signatures" on secured electronic record systems only.

The following describes the main documentation elements of patient/client management: 1) initial examination/evaluation, 2) visit/encounter, 3) reexamination, and 4) discharge or discontinuation summary.

### *Initial Examination/Evaluation*

Documentation of the initial encounter is typically called the "initial examination," "initial evaluation," or "initial examination/evaluation." Completion of the initial examination/ evaluation is typically completed in one visit, but may occur over more than one visit. Documentation elements for the initial examination/evaluation include the following:

Examination: Includes data obtained from the history, systems review, and tests and measures.

Evaluation: Evaluation is a thought process that may not include formal documentation. It may include documentation of the assessment of the data collected in the examination and identification of problems pertinent to patient/client management.

Diagnosis: Indicates level of impairment and functional limitation determined by the physical therapist. May be indicated by selecting one or more preferred practice patterns from the Guide to Physical Therapist Practice.

Prognosis: Provides documentation of the predictedlevel of improvement that might be attained through intervention and the amount of time required to reach that level. Prognosis is typically not a separate documentation elements, but the components are included as part of the plan of care.

Plan of care: Typically stated in general terms, includes goals, interventions planned, proposed frequency and duration, and discharge plans.

### Visit/Encounter

Documentation of a visit or encounter, often called a progress note or daily note, documents sequential implementation of the plan of care established by the physical therapist, including changes in patient/client status and variations and progressions of specific interventions used. Also may include specific plans for the next visit or visits.

### Reexamination

Documentation of reexamination includes data from repeated or new examination elements and is provided to evaluate progress and to modify or redirect intervention.

### Discharge or Discontinuation Summary

Documentation is required following conclusion of the current episode in the physical therapy intervention sequence, to summarize progression toward goals and discharge plans.

## General Guidelines

- Documentation is required for every visit/encounter.
- All documentation must comply with the applicable jurisdictional/regulatory requirements.
- All handwritten entries shall be made in ink and will include original signatures. Electronic entries are made with appropriate security and confidentiality provisions.
- Charting errors should be corrected by drawing a single line through the error and initialing and dating the chart or through the appropriate mechanism for electronic documentation that clearly indicates that a change was made without deletion of the original record.
- All documentation must include adequate identification of the patient/client and the physical therapist or physical therapist assistant:
  - The patient's/client's full name and identification number, if applicable, must be included on all official documents.
  - All entries must be dated and authenticated with the provider's full name and appropriate designation:
    - Documentation of examination, evaluation, diagnosis, prognosis, plan of care, and discharge summary must be authenticated by the physical therapist who provided the service.
    - Documentation of intervention in visit/encounter notes must be authenticated by the physical therapist or physical therapist assistant who provided the service.
    - Documentation by physical therapist or physical therapist assistant graduates or other physical therapists and physical therapist assistants pending receipt of an unrestricted license shall be authenticated by a licensed physical therapist, or, when permissible by law, documentation by physical therapist assistant graduates may be authenticated by a physical therapist assistant.
    - Documentation by students (SPT/SPTA) in physical therapist or physical therapist assistant programs must be additionally authenticated by the physical therapist or, when permissible by law, documentation by physical therapist assistant students may be authenticated by a physical therapist assistant.

- Documentation should include the referral mechanism by which physical therapy services are initiated. Examples include:
  - Self-referral/direct access
  - Request for consultation from another practitioner
- Documentation should include indication of no shows and cancellations.

# Initial Examination/Evaluation

### Examination (History, Systems Review, and Tests and Measures)

History:

Documentation of history may include the following:

- General demographics
- Social history
- Employment/work (Job/School/Play)
- Growth and development
- Living environment
- General health status (self-report, family report, caregiver report)
- Social/health habits (past and current)
- Family history
- Medical/surgical history
- Current condition(s)/Chief complaint(s)
- Functional status and activity level
- Medications
- Other clinical tests

Systems Review:

Documentation of systems review may include gathering data for the following systems:

- Cardiovascular/pulmonary
  - Blood Pressure
  - Edema
  - Heart Rate
  - Respiratory Rate
- Integumentary
  - Pliability (texture)
  - Presence of scar formation
  - Skin color
  - Skin integrity
- Musculoskeletal
  - Gross range of motion
  - Gross strength
  - Gross symmetry
  - Height
  - Weight
- Neuromuscular
  - Gross coordinated movement (eg, balance, locomotion, transfers, and transitions)
  - Motor function (motor control, motor learning)

Documentation of systems review may also address communication ability, affect, cognition, language, and learning style:

- Ability to make needs known
- Consciousness
- Expected emotional/behavioral responses
- Learning preferences (eg, *education needs, learning barriers*)
- Orientation (person, place, time)

Tests and Measures:
Documentation of tests and measures may include findings for the following categories:

- Aerobic Capacity/Endurance

    Examples of examination findings include:

    - Aerobic capacity during functional activities
    - Aerobic capacity during standardized exercise test protocols
    - Cardiovascular signs and symptoms in response to increased oxygen demand with exercise or activity
    - Pulmonary signs and symptoms in response to increased oxygen demand with exercise or activity

- Anthropometric Characteristics

    Examples of examination findings include:

    - Body composition
    - Body dimensions
    - Edema

- Arousal, attention, and cognition

    Examples of examination findings include:

    - Arousal and attention
    - Cognition
    - Communication
    - Consciousness
    - Motivation
    - Orientation to time, person, place, and situation
    - Recall

- Assistive and adaptive devices

    Examples of examination findings include:

    - Assistive or adaptive devices and equipment use during functional activities
    - Components, alignment, fit, and ability to care for the assistive or adaptive devices and equipment
    - Remediation of impairments, functional limitations, or disabilities with use of assistive or adaptive devices and equipment
    - Safety during use of assistive or adaptive devices and equipment

- Circulation (Arterial, Venous, Lymphatic)

    Examples of examination findings include:

    - Cardiovascular signs
    - Cardiovascular symptoms
    - Physiological responses to position change

- Cranial and Peripheral Nerve Integrity

    Examples of examination findings include:

    - Electrophysiological integrity
    - Motor distribution of the cranial nerves

- Motor distribution of the peripheral nerves
- Response to neural provocation
- Response to stimuli, including auditory, gustatory, olfactory, pharyngeal, vestibular, and visual
- Sensory distribution of the cranial nerves
- Sensory distribution of the peripheral nerves

- Environmental, Home, and Work (Job/School/Play) Barriers

  Examples of examination findings include:
  - Current and potential barriers
  - Physical space and environment

- Ergonomics and Body mechanics

  Examples of examination findings for *ergonomics* include:
  - Dexterity and coordination during work
  - Functional capacity and performance during work actions, tasks, or activities
  - Safety in work environments
  - Specific work conditions or activities
  - Tools, devices, equipment, and work-stations related to work actions, tasks, or activities

  Examples of examination findings for *body mechanics* include:
  - Body mechanics during self-care, home management, work, community, or leisure actions, tasks, or activities

- Gait, locomotion, and balance

  Examples of examination findings include:
  - Balance during functional activities with or without the use of assistive, adaptive, orthotic, protection, supportive, or prosthetic devices or equipment
  - Balance (dynamic and static) with or without the use of assistive, adaptive, orthotic, protective, supportive, or prosthetic devices or equipment
  - Gait and locomotion during functional activities with or without the use of assistive, adaptive, orthotic, protective, supportive, or prosthetic devices or equipment
  - Gait and locomotion with or without the use of assistive, adaptive, orthotic, protective, supportive, or prosthetic devices or equipment
  - Safety during gait, locomotion, and balance

- Integumentary Integrity

  Examples of examination findings include:

  *Associated skin*:
  - Activities, positioning, and postures that produce or relieve trauma to the skin
  - Assistive, adaptive, orthotic, protective, supportive, or prosthetic devices and equipment that may produce or relieve trauma to the skin
  - Skin characteristics

  *Wound*:
  - Activities, positioning, and postures that aggravate the wound or scar or that produce or relieve trauma
  - Burn
  - Signs of infection
  - Wound characteristics
  - Wound scar tissue characteristics

- Joint Integrity and Mobility

  Examples of examination findings include:
  - Joint integrity and mobility
  - Joint play movements
  - Specific body parts
- Motor Function

  Examples of examination findings include:
  - Dexterity, coordination, and agility
  - Electrophysiological integrity
  - Hand function
  - Initiation, modification, and control of movement patterns and voluntary postures
- Muscle Performance

  Examples of examination findings include:
  - Electrophysiological integrity
  - Muscle strength, power, and endurance
  - Muscle strength, power, and endurance during functional activities
  - Muscle tension
- Neuromotor development and sensory integration

  Examples of examination findings include:
  - Acquisition and evolution of motor skills
  - Oral motor function, phonation, and speech production
  - Sensorimotor integration
- Orthotic, protective, and supportive devices

  Examples of examination findings include:
  - Components, alignment, fit, and ability to care for the orthotic, protective, and supportive devices and equipment
  - Orthotic, protective, and supportive devices and equipment use during functional activities
  - Remediation of impairments, functional limitations, or disabilities with use of orthotic, protective, and supportive devices and equipment
  - Safety during use of orthotic, protective, and supportive devices and equipment
- Pain

  Examples of examination findings include:
  - Pain, soreness, and nocioception
  - Pain in specific body parts
- Posture

  Examples of examination findings include:
  - Postural alignment and position (dynamic)
  - Postural alignment and position (static)
  - Specific body parts
- Prosthetic requirements

  Examples of examination findings include:
  - Components, alignment, fit, and ability to care for prosthetic device
  - Prosthetic device use during functional activities
  - Remediation of impairments, functional limitations, or disabilities with use of the prosthetic device
  - Residual limb or adjacent segment
  - Safety during use of the prosthetic device

- Range of motion (including muscle length)
  - Examples of examination findings include:
  - Functional ROM
  - Joint active and passive movement
  - Muscle length, soft tissue extensibility, and flexibility
- Reflex integrity

  Examples of examination findings include:
  - Deep reflexes
  - Electrophysiological integrity
  - Postural reflexes and reactions, including righting, equilibrium, and protective reactions
  - Primitive reflexes and reactions
  - Resistance to passive stretch
  - Superficial reflexes and reactions
- Self-care and home management (including activities of daily living and instrumental activities of daily living)

  Examples of examination findings include:
  - Ability to gain access to home environments
  - Ability to perform self-care and home management activities with or without assistive, adaptive, orthotic, protective, supportive, or prosthetic devices and equipment
  - Safety in self-care and home management activities and environments
- Sensory integrity
  - Examples of examination findings include:
  - Combined/cortical sensations
  - Deep sensations
  - Electrophysiological integrity
- Ventilation and respiration

  Examples of examination findings include:
  - Pulmonary signs of respiration/gas exchange
  - Pulmonary signs of ventilatory function
  - Pulmonary symptoms
- Work (job/school/play), community, and leisure integration or reintegration (including instrumental activities of daily living)

  Examples of examination findings include:
  - Ability to assume or resume work (job/school/plan), community, and leisure activities with or without assistive, adaptive, orthotic, protective, supportive, or prosthetic devices and equipment
  - Ability to gain access to work (job/school/play), community, and leisure environments
  - Safety in work (job/school/play), community, and leisure activities and environments

## *Evaluation*

- Evaluation is a thought process that may not include formal documentation.However, the evaluation process may lead to documentation of impairments, functional limitations, and disabilities using formats such as:
  - A problem list
  - A statement of assessment of key factors (e.g., cognitive factors, co-morbidities, social support) influencing the patient/client status.

### Diagnosis

- Documentation of a diagnosis determined by the physical therapist may include impairment and functional limitations.

  Examples include:

  - Impaired Joint Mobility, Motor Function, Muscle Performance, and Range of Motion Associated With Localized Inflammation (4E)

  - Impaired Motor Function and Sensory Integrity Associated With Progressive Disorders of the Central Nervous System (5E)

  - Impaired Aerobic Capacity/Endurance Associated With Cardiovascular Pump Dysfunction or Failure (6D)

  - Impaired Integumentary Integrity Associated With Partial-Thickness Skin Involvement and Scar Formation (7C)

### Prognosis

- Documentation of the prognosis is typically included in the plan of care. See below.

### Plan of Care

- Documentation of the plan of care includes the following:

  - Overall goals stated in measurable terms that indicate the predicted level of improvement in function

  - A general statement of interventions to be used

  - Proposed duration and frequency of service required to reach the goals

  - Anticipated discharge plans

## Visit/Encounter

- Documentation of each visit/encounter shall include the following elements:

  - Patient/client self-report (as appropriate).

  - Identification of specific interventions provided, including frequency, intensity, and duration as appropriate. Examples include:

  - Knee extension, three sets, ten repetitions, 10# weight

  - Transfer training bed to chair with sliding board

  - Equipment provided

  - Changes in patient/client impairment, functional limitation, and disability status as they relate to the plan of care.

- Response to interventions, including adverse reactions, if any.

- Factors that modify frequency or intensity of intervention and progression goals, including patient/client adherence to patient/client-related instructions.

- Communication/consultation with providers/patient/client/family/ significant other.

- Documentation to plan for ongoing provision of services for the next visit(s), which is suggested to include, but not be limited to:

  - The interventions with objectives

  - Progression parameters

  - Precautions, if indicated

### Reexamination

- Documentation of reexamination shall include the following elements:

  - Documentation of selected components of examination to update patient's/client's impairment, function, and/or disability status.

  - Interpretation of findings and, when indicated, revision of goals.

  - When indicated, revision of plan of care, as directly correlated with goals as documented.

## Discharge/Discontinuation Summary

- Documentation of discharge or discontinuation shall include the following elements:

  - Current physical/functional status.

  - Degree of goals achieved and reasons for goals not being achieved.

  - Discharge/discontinuation plan related to the patient/client's continuing care.
    Examples include:

  - Home program.

  - Referrals for additional services.

  - Recommendations for follow-up physical therapy care.

  - Family and caregiver training.

  - Equipment provided.

Reprinted with permission from the American Physical Therapy Association. http://www.apta.org/AM/Template.cfm?Section=Home&TEMPLATE=/CM/ContentDisplay.cfm&CONTENTID=31688 Accessed on December 11, 2007.

# Appendix B: Abbreviations and Symbols

This list provides many of the abbreviations and symbols used in medical charts and in physical therapy records. You should check with your facility regarding abbreviations and symbols that are "approved" for use, because they can vary. Also, note that some abbreviations have more than one meaning. Be careful and understand the context in which each abbreviation is used.

**A**

| | |
|---|---|
| abdominal | abd |
| abduction | abd |
| abductor digiti minimi | ADM |
| abductor pollicus brevis | APB |
| abductor pollicus longus | APL |
| above elbow | AE |
| above knee | AK |
| accuracy | acc |
| acetylcholine | Ach |
| acid-fast bacilli | AFB |
| active assistive range of motion | AAROM |
| active range of motion | AROM |
| activities of daily living | ADL |
| acute lymphoblastic leukemia | ALL |
| acute myeloblastic leukemia | AML |
| acute renal failure | ARF |
| adduction | add |
| adrenocorticotropic hormone | ACTH |
| adult (acute) respiratory distress syndrome | ARDS |
| Advance Beneficiary Notice | ABN |
| after meals | pc |
| after noon | pm |
| against medical advice | AMA |
| ambulatory or ambulates | AMB |
| Americans with Disabilities Act | ADA |
| amount | amt |
| ampere | A |
| amyotrophic lateral sclerosis (Lou Gehrig's Disease) | ALS |
| analysis of variance | ANOVA |
| angiotensin-converting enzyme | ACE |
| ankle foot orthosis | AFO |
| ankle pump (or anterior-posterior) | AP |
| anterior cruciate ligament | ACL |
| anterior talofibular | ATF |
| anterior-posterior | AP or A/P |
| antibody | Ab |
| antigen | Ag |
| aortic component of second heart sound | A2 |
| appropriate for gestational age | AGA |
| approximate | approx |
| arterial blood gas(es) | ABG(s) |
| atreriosclerotic cardiovascular disease | ASCVD |
| arteriosclerotic heart disease | ASHD |
| as desired | ad lib |
| as needed | PRN |
| assistive/augmentative communication | AAC |
| as soon as possible | ASAP |

| | |
|---|---|
| aspiration | asp |
| aspirin | ASA |
| assessment | A: |
| assistive device; Alzheimer's Disease | AD |
| at bedtime | n.s. |
| atrial fibrillation | AF |
| atrial septal defect | ASD |
| atriovenous or atrioventricular | AV |
| attention | atten. or ATTN: |
| audiovisual | A-V |
| auditory | aud. |
| auscultation and percussion | A & P |
| autoimmune deficiency syndrome | AIDS |

**B**

| | |
|---|---|
| barium | Ba |
| bathroom privileges | BRP or B.R.P. |
| beats per minute | BPM or bpm |
| Beck Depression Inventory, 2nd edition | BDI-II |
| before meals | ac |
| before noon | am |
| below elbow | BE |
| below knee | BK |
| benign prostatic hypertrophy | BPH |
| bilateral lower extremities | BLE |
| biopsy | Bx |
| blood brain barrier | BBB |
| blood pressure | BP |
| blood urea nitrogen | BUN |
| body mass index | BMI |
| body surface area | BSA |
| bone conduction | B/C |
| bone mineral density | BMD |
| bowel movement | BM |
| brain injury | BI |
| by mouth | po |

**C**

| | |
|---|---|
| calcaneofibular | CF |
| calcium | Ca |
| calorie | cal |
| cancel (or crutches) | cx |
| cancer or carcinoma | CA |
| carbohydrate | CHO or CARB |
| carbon dioxide | $CO_2$ |
| cardiomyopathy | CMP |

| | | | |
|---|---|---|---|
| cardiopulmonary resuscitation | CPR | distal radioulnar joint | DRUJ |
| cardiovascular | CV | do not resuscitate | DNR |
| carpometacarpal | CMC | doctor of chiropractic; chiropractor | DC |
| Center for Disease Control | CDC | doctor of osteopath | DO |
| Center for Medicare and Medicaid | | dorsal interossei | DI |
| Services | CMS | dorsiflexion | DF |
| centimeter | cm | durable medical equipment | DME |
| central line placement | CLP | | |
| central nervous system | CNS | **E** | |
| cerebral palsy | CP or C.P. | each | ea. |
| cerebrospinal fluid | CSF | eating intervention program | EIP |
| cerebrovascular accident | CVA | effect size | ES |
| cervical (vertebrae) | C | elbow orthosis | EO |
| (*followed by 1, 2, ...etc.*) | | electrocardiogram | EKG, ECG |
| certified occupational therapist assistant | COTA | electroencephalogram | EEG |
| certified registered nurse practitioner | CRNP | electromyogram | EMG |
| chief complaint | c/c, C/C, | electronystagmograph | ENG |
| | or C.C. | electrophysiological stimulation | EPS |
| chlorine | Cl | emergency medical services | EMS |
| chronic obstructive pulmonary disease | COPD | endotracheal | E-T |
| closed head injury | CHI | endotracheal tube | ET tube |
| clostridium difficile | C-diff | end-stage renal disease | ESRD |
| cold whirlpool | CWP | erythrocyte sedimentation rate | ESR |
| Common Procedural Terminology | CPT | Escherichia coli | E. coli |
| complains of | c/o or C/O | esophagogastroduodenoscopy | EGD |
| complete blood count | CBC | ethyl alcohol | EtOH or |
| computed tomography | CT | | ETOH |
| computerized axial tomography | CAT | evaluation | eval |
| congestive heart failure | CHF | evidence-based practice | EBP |
| contact guard assist | CGA | eversion | ev, ever |
| continue | cont. | every | q |
| continuous passive motion | CPM | every eight hours | q8h |
| continuous positive airway pressure | CPAP | every four hours | q4h |
| contralateral | c/l | every hour | qh |
| coronary artery bypass graft | CABG | every morning | qam |
| coronary artery disease | CAD | every other day | qod |
| coronary or critical care unit | CCU | every three hours | q3h |
| creatinine phosphokinase | CPK | every two hours | q2h |
| crutches (or cancel) | cx | exercise | ex. or ex |
| cubic centimeter | cc or cm$^3$ | expiratory reserve volume | ERV |
| culture and sensitivity | C & S | extensor carpi radialis brevis | ECRB |
| cytomegalovirus | CMV | extensor carpi radialis longus | ECRL |
| | | extensor carpi ulnaris | ECU |
| | | extensor digiti minimi | EDM |
| **D** | | extensor digitorum communis | EDC |
| date of injury | DOI | extensor indicis proprius | EIP |
| deep brain stimulator | DBS | extensor pollicus brevis | EPB |
| deep tendon reflex | DTR | extensor pollicus longus | EPL |
| deep vein thrombosis | DVT | extracellular fluid | ECF |
| degenerative disc disease | DDD | eyes, ears, nose, and throat | EENT |
| degenerative joint disease | DJD | | |
| department | dept. | | |
| dependent | dep. | **F** | |
| developmental delay | DD | fair (manual muscle test) | 3/5 |
| Diabetes Mellitus | DM | family history | FH |
| diagnosis | dx | fasting blood sugar | FBS |
| diagnosis related group | DRG | Federation of State Boards of Physical | |
| differential | diff | Therapy | FSBPT |
| Disabilities of the Arm, Shoulder, | | fetal heart rate | FHR |
| and Hand (outcome measure) | DASH | fever of unknown origin | FUO |
| discharge or discontinue | d/c | Fibromyalgia Syndrome | FM |
| distal interphalangeal (joint) | DIP(J) | flexor carpi radialis | FCR |

| | | | |
|---|---|---|---|
| flexor carpi ulnaris | FCU | human immunodeficiency virus | HIV |
| flexor digiti minimi | FDM | hypertension | HTN |
| flexor digitorum profundus | FDP | | |
| flexor digitorum superficialis | FDS | **I** | |
| flexor pollicus brevis | FPB | immediately | stat |
| flexor pollicus longus | FPL | immunoglobulin | Ig |
| fluid | fl | incision and drainage | I & D |
| Food and Drug Administration | FDA | Individuals with Disabilities in | |
| follow up | F/U or f/u | Education Act | IDEA |
| foot orthosis | FO | in-patient | IP |
| forced expiratory volume | FEV | in-patient rehabilitation facility | IRF |
| forced vital capacity | FVC | inspiratory capacity | IC |
| four times a day | qid | inspiratory reserve volume | IRV |
| fracture | fx or Fx | instrumental activities of daily living | IADL |
| frequency | fo | insulin-dependent diabetes mellitus | IDDM |
| front wheeled walker | FFW | intake and output | I & O |
| full thickness skin graft | FTSG | intensive care unit | ICU |
| full weight bearing | FWB | *International Classification of Disease,* | |
| functional capacity evaluation | FCE | *Ninth Revision* | ICD-9 |
| functional electrical stimulation | FES | *International Classification of Disease,* | |
| functional independence measure | FIM | *Tenth Revision* | ICD-10 |
| functional outcome report | FOR | *International Classification of* | |
| functional residual capacity | FRC | *Functioning, Disability, and Health* | ICF |
| | | *International Classification of Health* | |
| **G** | | *Interventions* | ICHI |
| gastroesophageal reflux disease | GERD | *International Classification of* | |
| gastrointestinal | GI | *Impairments, Disabilities, and Handicaps* | ICIDH |
| gestational age | GA | interphalangeal | IP |
| glenohumeral | GH | intraclass correlation coefficient | ICC |
| glucose tolerance test | GTT | intracranial pressure | ICP |
| gluteal sets | GS | intramuscular | IM |
| good (manual muscle test) | 4/5 | intravenous | IV |
| gram | g | inversion | inv |
| | | isoniazid | INH |
| **H** | | | |
| hand orthosis (or hip orthosis) | HO | **J** | |
| hand rail | HR | Joint Commission on Accreditation of | |
| head of bed | HOB | Health Care Organizations | JCAHO |
| Health Care Financing Administration | HCFA | | |
| Health Insurance Portability and | | **K** | |
| Accountability Act | HIPAA | kilogram | kg |
| health maintenance organization | HMO | knee ankle foot orthosis | KAFO |
| heart rate | HR | | |
| hematocrit | Hct | **L** | |
| hemoglobin | Hb | lateral collateral ligament | LCL |
| hemoglobin and hematocrit | H & H | left hand dominant | LHD |
| hepatitis B virus | HBV | lifestyle | L/S, l/s |
| hepatitis A virus | HAV | liter | L |
| hepatitis C virus | HCV | long arc quadriceps exercise | LAQ |
| herniated nucleus pulposus | HNP | long arm cast | LAC |
| hertz | Hz | long leg cast | LLC |
| high-density lipoprotein | HDL | long term functional goal | LTFG |
| hip orthosis (or hand orthosis) | HO | long term goal | LTG |
| history | hx | low-density lipoprotein | LDL |
| history and physical | H & P | lower motor neuron | LMN |
| history of | h/o | lumbar puncture | LP |
| history of present illness | HPI | lunotriquetral | LT |
| home exercise program | HEP | | |
| hormone replacement therapy | HRT | **M** | |
| hot pack | HP | magnetic resonance image | MRI |
| hour | h or hr | manual muscle test | MMT |

| mechanism of injury | MOI |
| medial collateral ligament | MCL |
| medicines, medications | MED(S) |
| megahertz | MHz |
| metacarpophalangeal | MCP |
| metatarsophalangeal | MTP |
| meter | m |
| methicillin-resistant *Staphylococcus aureus* | MRSA |
| millimeter | mm |
| millimeters of mercury | mm Hg |
| millivolt | mV |
| minimal clinical important difference | MCID |
| minimal detectable change | MDC |
| Minimum Data Set | MDS |
| months | mos |
| multi-infarct dementia | MID |
| Multiple Sclerosis | MS |
| muscle | m. |
| Muscular Dystrophy | MD |
| Myasthenia Gravis | MG |
| myocardial infarction | MI |

**N**

| narrow base quad cane | NBQC |
| National Center for Medical Rehabilitation Research | NCMRR |
| nausea and vomiting | n & v |
| neonatal intensive care unit | NICU |
| nerve | n. |
| neurodevelopmental treatment | NDT |
| neuromuscular electrical stimulation | NMES |
| newton | N |
| non-insulin dependent diabetes mellitus | NIDDM |
| non-steroidal anti-inflammatory drug(s) | NSAID(S) |
| non-weight bearing | NWB |
| normal (manual muscle test) | 5/5 |
| not applicable | N/A |
| not tested | NT |
| nothing by mouth | NPO |
| nothing by mouth | NPO |
| Notice of Exclusion of Medicare Benefits | NEMB |

**O**

| objective | O: |
| obsessive compulsive disorder | OCD |
| obstetrics and gynecology | OB/GYN |
| Occupational Safety and Health Administration | OSHA |
| occupational therapist | OT |
| occupational therapist registered and licensed | OTR/L |
| open reduction internal fixation | ORIF |
| operating room | OR |
| opponens digiti minimi | ODM |
| opponens pollicus | OP |
| organic brain syndrome | OBS |
| osteoarthritis | OA |
| Osteogenesis Imperfecta | OI |
| ounce | oz |

| Outcome and Assessment Information Set | OASIS |
| out of bed | OOB |
| outpatient | OP |
| over-the-counter (ie, drugs) | OTC |
| oxygen | $O_2$ or O2 |
| oxygen saturation | $SaO_2$ |

**P**

| palmar interossei | PI |
| palmaris longus | PL |
| Parkinson's Disease | PD |
| partial thromboplastin time | PTT |
| partial weight bearing (usually 50% unless otherwise indicated; may need to check with physician to clarify) | PWB |
| passive range of motion | PROM |
| past medical history | PMH |
| patient | pt. or Pt. |
| patient-controlled anesthesia | PCA |
| percutaneous endoscopic gastrostomy (tube) | PEG |
| percutaneous transluminal coronary angioplasty | PTCA |
| peripheral nervous system | PNS |
| peripheral vascular disease | PVD |
| physical therapist | PT |
| physical therapist assistant | PTA |
| physician | MD |
| physician assistant | PA-C |
| Physicians' Desk Reference | PDR |
| plan | P: |
| plantarflexion | PF |
| poor (manual muscle test) | 2/5 |
| positron emission tomography | PET |
| post operative | post op |
| posterior cruciate ligament | PCL |
| posterior talofibular | PTF |
| posterior-anterior | PA |
| potassium | K |
| preferred provider organization | PPO |
| prescription | Rx |
| primary care provider | PCP |
| prior to admission | PTA |
| probability of success | p |
| problem | Pr: |
| problem-oriented medical record | POMR |
| pronator quadratus | PQ |
| pronator teres | PT |
| proprioceptive neuromuscular facilitation | PNF |
| Prospective Payment System | PPS |
| protected health information | PHI |
| prothrombin time | PT |
| proximal interphalangeal | PIP |
| proximal radioulnar joint | PRUJ |
| pulmonary embolism | PE |
| pulmonary function test | PFT |
| pupils equal, round (regular), reactive to light, and accommodating | PERRLA |

**Q**

| | |
|---|---|
| quad set/quadriceps set | QS |

**R**

| | |
|---|---|
| radial collateral ligament | RCL |
| radial deviation | RD |
| radiocarpal | RC |
| range of motion | ROM |
| rate of perceived exertion | RPE |
| reciprocating gait orthosis | RGO |
| red blood cell | RBC |
| repetitions | reps |
| reschedule | r/s |
| residual volume | RV |
| Resource Utilization Group | RUG |
| respiratory distress syndrome | RDS |
| respiratory rate | RR |
| return to clinic | RTC |
| return to work | RTW |
| review of systems | ROS |
| rheumatoid arthritis | RA |
| right hand dominant | RHD |
| rule out | r/o; R/O |

**S**

| | |
|---|---|
| scapholunate | SL |
| scapulothoracic | ST |
| short arc quadriceps exercise | SAQ |
| short arm cast | SAC |
| short leg cast | SLC |
| short term goal | STG |
| shortness of breath | SOB |
| short-term memory | STM |
| shoulder orthosis | SO |
| side lying | SL |
| skilled nursing facility | SNF |
| sodium | Na |
| speech language pathologist | SLP |
| spinal cord injury | SCI |
| Spinal Muscular Atrophy | SMA |
| split thickness skin graft | STSG |
| stand by assist | SBA |
| standard error of the measurement | SEM |
| standardized response mean | SRM |
| status post | s/p |
| straight leg raise | SLR |
| student physical therapist | SPT |
| student physical therapist assistant | SPTA |
| subjective | S: |
| sudden infant death syndrome | SIDS |
| supervision | s or SVN |
| Systemic Lupus Erythmatosus | SLE |

**T**

| | |
|---|---|
| tablespoon | tbsp or T |
| teaspoon | tsp or t |
| temperature | T |
| tempromandibular joint | TMJ |
| tender to palpation | TTP |
| terminal knee extension | TKE |
| therapeutic activity | TA |
| therapeutic procedure | TP |
| three times a day | tid |
| tidal volume | TV |
| times | x (i.e. 3x/ week) |
| toe touch weight bearing | TTWB |
| total hip arthroplasy | THA |
| total hip replacement | THR |
| total knee arthroplasy | TKA |
| total knee replacement | TKR |
| total parenteral nutrition | TPN |
| trace (manual muscle test) | 1/5 |
| traction (or treatment) | tx |
| transient ischemic attack | TIA |
| traumatic brain injury | TBI |
| treatment (or traction) | tx |
| triangular fibrocartilagenous complex | TFCC |
| tuberculosis | TB |
| twice a day | bid or b.i.d. |

**U**

| | |
|---|---|
| ulnar collateral ligament | UCL |
| ulnar deviation | UD |
| ultrasound | US |
| ultraviolet | UV |
| upper motor neuron | UMN |
| urinary tract infection | UTI |

**V**

| | |
|---|---|
| volt | V |

**W**

| | |
|---|---|
| warm whirlpool | WWP |
| water | $H_2O$ |
| watt | W |
| watts per centimeters squared | $w/cm^2$ |
| week | wk |
| weight bearing as tolerated | WBAT |
| wheelchair | w/c |
| whirlpool | WP |
| white blood cell | WBC |
| wide base quad cane | WBQC |
| within functional limits | WFL |
| within normal limits | WNL |
| World Health Organization | WHO |
| World Health Organization–Family of International Classifications | WHO-FIC |
| wrist hand finger orthosis | WHFO |
| wrist hand orthosis | WHO |

# Common Symbols

| | |
|---|---|
| about | ~ |
| after | $\bar{p}$ |
| ascend or increase | ↑ |
| assist (min, mod, max assist) | a, (A), or ⓐ |
| at | @ |
| before | $\bar{a}$ |
| both or bilateral | B, (B), o ⓑ |
| degrees | ° |
| degrees Celsius | ° C |
| degrees Fahrenheit | ° F |
| dependent | D, (D), or ⓓ |
| descend or decrease | ↓ |
| equal, equal to | = |
| extension | / |
| female | ♀ |
| for, except | $\bar{x}$ |
| greater than, greater than or equal to | >, ≥ |

| | |
|---|---|
| hour, foot | ′ |
| inch, minute | ″ |
| independent | I, (I), or Ⓚ |
| left | L, (L), or Ⓛ |
| less than, less than or equal to | <, ≤ |
| male | ♂ |
| micro | μ |
| negative | -, (-), or ⊖ |
| not equal to, unequal | ≠ |
| number of individuals assisting (one, two) | x1, x2 |
| parallel bars | // |
| per | / |
| positive | + |
| possible, question, suggestive | ? |
| pounds | # or lbs. |
| primary | 1° |
| right | R, (R), or Ⓡ |
| secondary, secondary to | 2°, 2° to |
| with | $\bar{c}$ |
| without | $\bar{s}$ |

# Appendix C: Sample Forms

# Physical Therapy Examination

Patient's Name_____ Age_____ Date of Examination_____
Referred by:_____ for:_____
Medical Diagnosis_____ DOI/Onset_____
Affected side: ❑ Right   ❑ Left   ❑ Both             Hand Dominance: ❑ Right    ❑ Left
Gender: ❑ Male   ❑ Female
**History:**
History of Present Illness (HPI):_____
_____
_____
Chief complaint:_____
Hx of similar problem ❑ No   ❑ Yes, describe: _____
PMH/Co-morbidities/Complexities: ❑ None    ❑ Yes _____
_____
Surgical history ❑ None   ❑ Yes _____
Significant family history: ❑ None  ❑ Yes _____
Current services being received for this problem: ❑   None ❑ Yes _____
Prior treatment for this problem (including PT): ❑ None  ❑ Yes _____
Medications: ❑ None  ❑ Yes (include dosage)_____
Drug allergies: ❑ None  ❑ Yes _____
Imaging Studies for present problem: ❑ None  ❑ Yes _____
Orthotic/assistive/ prosthetic devices ❑ None  ❑ Yes _____

**For chronic conditions:** Recent change in status:_____
Date of change/decline:_____ New safety issues:_____
Functional level before change:_____
_____

**Living Environment/Situation:**_____
Available social support:_____
Requires Assistance: ❑ No ❑ Yes _____
Obstacles: ❑ No ❑ Yes _____
General health/health habits:_____
     ❑ See attached general health questionnaire
Current/Prior Functional Status: ADLs: _____
     Home management tasks: _____
     Community tasks: _____
     Occupation/Work status/School:_____
       Requirements:_____
     Recreation/Leisure: _____
     Global Rating (0-100%):_____
    ❑ See attached self-report disability/functional questionnaire

Patient's Therapy Goals:_____

Need for PT: ❑ Return to PLOF     ❑ Decrease assistance currently required
　　　　　　　 ❑ Change in living environment

Patient concerns:_____

**Pain:** Verbal rating (0-10):_____ Description:_____

Frequency/Duration of Pain: _____

Activities that: increase pain: _____ decrease pain:_____

Numbness/Tingling ❑ None ❑ Yes, Location: _____

Temperature changes ❑ None ❑ Yes, Location: _____

**Gross Review of Systems:**

Cardiopulmonary:　　　BP_____ HR_____ RR_____ O$_2$ sat_____
　　　　　　　　　　　 ❑ Not impaired ❑ Impaired _____
　　　　　　　　　　　 ❑ (see specific exam below)

Integumentary:　　　　 ❑ Not impaired ❑ Impaired _____
　　　　　　　　　　　 ❑ (see specific exam below)

Musculoskeletal:　　　　❑ Not impaired　❑ Impaired _____
　　　　　　　　　　　 ❑ (see specific exam below)

Neurological:　　　　　 ❑ Not impaired　❑ Impaired _____
　　　　　　　　　　　 ❑ (see specific exam below)

Cognitive/Communicative Ability: ❑ Not impaired　❑ Impaired _____

**Physical Therapy Tests/Measures:**

(identify/list those done frequently)


(include impairments and function)


(include space for "Other")


Functional assessment(s): ❑ See attached functional assessment [NDI, Oswestry, DASH, PRWE, SF-36, FIM, etc]


**Today's Interventions:**

Collaboration/Communication: ❑ None　❑ Yes_____

HEP Instructions: _____
_____

Other Pt. Education: _____
_____

　　　Pt./caregiver response to teaching: _____

Procedural Interventions: _____
_____
_____
_____

# Physical Therapy Assessment and Plan of Care

Patient Name: _____ Patient's DOB:_____ PT Examination Date_____

---

**\*\*For the physician**

I have read and concur with the plan of care written below for this patient:

_____     _____     _____

Name of Supervising Physician     Physician Signature     Date

---

Summary/Comments:_____

_____

Primary Medical Diagnosis: _____ (ICD-9):_____ PT Diagnosis:_____

Co-morbidities influencing treatment (and ICD-9):_____

Patient's Rehab Potential: _____

Skilled services required for: _____["addressing the following impairments and functional

limitations"] _____

Problem List:

| Physical therapy impairments: | Functional problems: (Include ADL, home management, community, work, leisure) |
|---|---|
| 1. | 1. |
| 2. | 2. |
| 3. | 3. |
| 4. | 4. |
| 5. | 5. |

Expected Outcomes (to be met by_____):

     A.

     B.

     C.

     D.

     E.

STGs  (to be met by_____):

     A-1.

     B-1.

     C-1.

     D-1.

     E-1.

**Treatment Plan:**    Frequency/Duration services will be provided: _____

Physical therapy modality/procedure code(s)

| 1. | 4. |
|---|---|
| 2. | 5. |
| 3. | 6. |

☐   The  patient/care giver is in agreement with the plan.

Examination, assessment, and plan of care completed and written by: _____

                                                      (PT Signature)

## References

1. American Physical Therapy Association. Guide to Physical Therapist Practice, 2nd ed. Alexandria, VA: APTA; 2001
2. Centers for Medicare and Medicaid Services, Medicare Benefit Policy Manual, Chapter 15, Section 220

# Treatment Encounter Note #_____

Patient Name_____ Date_____

Subjective Report_____
_____
_____
_____
_____

Objective Measurements _____
_____
_____
_____
_____
_____

Interventions (communication, education, and procedural interventions):




_____ Total timed code minutes          _____ Total treatment time

Response to treatment_____
_____
_____

Change(s) in status since initial visit _____
_____
_____

Factors warranting change to plan of care_____
_____
_____

Plans for next visit_____
_____

Signature(s)_____

# Progress Report

Patient Name _____   Treatment interval _____

Date Progress Report written____

Subjective Report_____

_____

_____

Objective Measurements _____

_____

_____

_____

_____

| Current Outcome Goals to be met by_____ | Progress toward goals: |
|---|---|
| A. | |
| B. | |
| C. | |
| D. | |
| E. | |
| F. | |

Changes to goals or plan of care and rationale:_____

_____

_____

Overall assessment of progress:_____

_____

Plans for further interventions:_____

_____

_____

_____

_____

Physical Therapist

For the physician:

I have read and concur with the plan of care for this patient.

_____

Name of Supervising Physician        Physician Signature                        Date

# Appendix D: Preferred Practice Patterns

## Musculoskeletal

Pattern A:    Primary Prevention/Risk Reduction for Skeletal Demineralization

Pattern B:    Impaired Posture

Pattern C:    Impaired Muscle Performance

Pattern D:    Impaired Joint Mobility, Motor Function, Muscle Performance, and Range of Motion Associated With Connective Tissue Dysfunction

Pattern E:    Impaired Joint Mobility, Motor Function, Muscle Performance, and Range of Motion Associated With Localized Inflammation

Pattern F:    Impaired Joint Mobility, Motor Function, Muscle Performance, Range of Motion, and Reflex Integrity Associated With Spinal Disorders

Pattern G:    Impaired Joint Mobility, Motor Function, Muscle Performance, and Range of Motion Associated With Fracture

Pattern H:    Impaired Joint Mobility, Motor Function, Muscle Performance, and Range of Motion Associated With Joint Arthroplasty

Pattern I:    Impaired Joint Mobility, Motor Function, Muscle Performance, and Range of Motion Associated With Bony or Soft Tissue Surgery

Pattern J:    Impaired Joint Mobility, Motor Function, Muscle Performance, and Range of Motion, Gait, Locomotion, and Balance Associated With Amputation

## Neuromuscular

Pattern A:    Primary Prevention/Risk Reduction for Loss of Balance and Falling

Pattern B:    Impaired Neuromotor Development

Pattern C:    Impaired Motor Function and Sensory Integrity Associated With Nonprogressive Disorders of the Central Nervous System – Congenital Origin or Acquired in Infancy or Childhood

Pattern D:    Impaired Motor Function and Sensory Integrity Associated With Nonprogressive Disorders of the Central Nervous System – Acquired in Adolescence of Adulthood

Pattern E:    Impaired Motor Function and Sensory Integrity Associated With Progressive Disorders of the Central Nervous System

Pattern F:    Impaired Peripheral Nerve Integrity and Muscle Performance Associated With Peripheral Nerve Injury

Pattern G:    Impaired Motor Function and Sensory Integrity Associated With Acute or Chronic Polyneuropathies

Pattern H:    Impaired Motor Function, Peripheral Nerve Integrity, and Sensory Integrity Associated with Nonprogressive Disorders of the Spinal Cord

Pattern I:    Impaired Arousal, Range of Motion, and Motor Control Associated With Coma, Near Coma, or Vegetative State

## Cardiovascular/Pulmonary

Pattern A:    Primary Prevention/Risk Reduction for Cardiovascular/Pulmonary Disorders

Pattern B:    Impaired Aerobic Capacity/Endurance Associated With Deconditioning

Pattern C:    Impaired Ventilation, Respiration/Gas Exchange, and Aerobic Capacity/Endurance Associated With Airway Clearance Dysfunction

Pattern D:    Impaired Aerobic Capacity/Endurance Associated With Cardiovascular Pump Dysfunction or Failure

Pattern E:   Impaired Ventilation and Respiration/Gas Exchange Associated with Ventilatory Pump Dysfunction or Failure

Pattern F:   Impaired Ventilation and Respiration/Gas Exchange Associated with Respiratory Failure

Pattern G:   Impaired Ventilation, Respiration/Gas Exchange, and Aerobic Capacity/Endurance Associated with Respiratory Failure in the Neonate

Pattern H:   Impaired Circulation and Anthropometric Dimensions Associated With Lymphatic System Disorders

# Integumentary

Pattern A:   Primary Prevention/Risk Reduction for Integumentary Disorders

Pattern B:   Impaired Integumentary Integrity Associated With Superficial Skin Involvement

Pattern C:   Impaired Integumentary Integrity Associated With Partial-Thickness Skin Involvement and Scar Formation

Pattern D:   Impaired Integumentary Integrity Associated With Full-Thickness Involvement and Scar Formation

Pattern E:   Impaired Integumentary Integrity Associated With Skin Involvement Extending Into Fascia, Muscle, or Bone and Scar Formation

From *The Guide to Physical Therapist Practice*. Alexandria, VA: APTA; 2001.

# Glossary

**Abuse**: Billing or requesting payment for items that are not covered by a third-party payer or misusing billing codes. Usually a result of an error, or unawareness of the proper code(s) or coding procedure(s).

**Activities of daily living (ADL)**: Skills required to be independent in day-to-day living, eg, bathing, grooming, self-care, mobility, toileting, transfers, etc.

**Activity**: Completion of a task or action by an individual.

**Activity limitation**: Difficulties or limitations encountered by an individual who is attempting to complete a task or carry out an activity.

**Addendum**: An entry made into the medical record that adds new information to a already existing note that is completed and signed; Follows the original documentation without skipping lines and is titled, "Addendum:".

**Advance Beneficiary Notice (ABN)**: A form or notice that a health care provider asks a Medicare beneficiary to sign when providing a service that may not be covered by Medicare. In signing the ABN, the Medicare beneficiary agrees to pay for the service if it is not covered by Medicare (see also Notice of Exclusion of Medicare Benefits).

**Assessment**: The physical therapist's clinical judgment or overall impression of the patient; The A: section of a SOAP note; In the SOAP note, includes a brief patient summary, rehab potential, medical and/or PT diagnosis, expected goals and potential for achievement; may also include patient progress or regression, status toward existing goals, overall improvement, or justification/need for skilled services.

**Attribute**: A variable; A characteristic or quality that is measured.

**Auditor**: A person who checks accounts of an individual, group, or organization. An auditor for an insurance company may review a provider's records to determine if services that were provided to a patient are consistent with what was billed.

**Authenticate**: A process that verifies a note is complete, genuine, and accurate; Usually done in the form of applying the signature of the individual writing the note.

**Capacity**: Extent of an activity limitation; Direct manifestations of the health state including activities performed without assistance; Scored in Activities and Participation Domain for ICF evaluation scheme.

**Carrier**: A privately run insurance company that contracts with the government to pay bills for Medicare Part B. Carriers are determined by geographic region and can be found at http://www.cms.hhs.gov/contacts/incardir.asp#4.

**Case-mix group**: Categorization or grouping of patients who are admitted to hospitals or other facilities according to common characteristics such as diagnosis, disease, and functional status.

**Centers for Medicare and Medicaid Services (CMS)**: A federal government agency that administers Medicare and works with state governments to administer Medicaid and State Children's Health Insurance Programs (SCHIP). CMS is housed within the Department of Health and Human Services (www.cms.hhs.gov).

**Claim**: The process of submitting a bill to an insurance company; may be made by the patient or the health care provider, depending on the insurance plan.

**Coding**: The process of assigning codes to describe a patient's health care problem and/or the services rendered.

**Co-morbidity (or co-morbidities)**: Aspect(s) of the patient's past medical history that affect(s) his or her current episode of care; or, a previous or current medical condition that has the potential to hinder or slow progress in physical therapy.

**Common Procedural Terminology (CPT)**: A system for coding procedures provided to patients. The CPT coding system was developed by the American Medical Association, which regularly updates the codes to reflect current practice.

**Compliance**: The ongoing process of keeping current on laws, regulations, and policies impacting the delivery and payment for health care services and practicing within those laws, regulations, and policies.

**Copayment**: Many health insurance plans require a patient to pay a portion of the cost of services provided; this portion is referred to as a copayment. For example, a patient is covered by a health insurance plan that requires the patient pay a $20 copayment for each physical therapy visit. For each visit, the patient pays $20; the insurance plan pays the remainder of the charge for the visit.

**Cronbach's alpha (α)**: A reliability value given as a measure internal consistency.

**Deductible**: A term used to refer to the amount a patient must pay before his/her insurance will take over payment. For instance, if a patient is covered by an insurance plan with a $500 deductible, the patient is responsible for paying the first $500 of care provided during a year. After reaching the $500 deductible, the patient's insurance plan will begin paying for covered health care services.

**Diagnosis (Dx)**: A medical diagnosis, assigned by the physician, which identifies the injury, illness, or disease, usually at the cellular, organ, or system level. A physical therapy diagnosis, assigned by the physical therapist, identifies the impact of the patient's medical diagnosis and impairments on movement and function.

**Diagnosis-related group (DRG)**: A categorization system used to group patients according to his or her diagnosis, treatment, age, and other relevant criteria. DRGs are used as part of the inpatient prospective payment system.

**Dictation**: Providing verbal communication that is later transcribed (copied into written text).

**Disability**: The inability or limitation in performing socially defined roles and/or tasks that would normally be expected of an individual within a given culture and/or environment.

**Disablement**: The consequences of disease as it pertains to the relationship between body structures, ability to carry out tasks, and ability to function within society.

**Disablement Framework**: A model or guide used to organize disability-related terminology and concepts.

**Discharge (D/C)**: Terminating care provided to a patient at the end of an episode of care when expected goals have been achieved.

**Discharge summary**: Part of the physical therapy documentation; Written at the end of an episode of care, when the patient is discharged from a facility or provider, or when physical therapy services are discontinued; Summarizes the care provided, patient progress, and final outcome.

**Discontinuation**: A process described in *The Guide to Physical Therapist Practice* as the termination of services during a single episode of care when: 1) a patient/family member/caregiver declines or refuses further interventions; 2) a patient cannot meet the expected goals due to medical, psychosocial, or financial reasons; or (3) a physical therapist feels the patient will no longer benefit.

**Documentation**: A record of Patient/Client Management during an episode of care.

**Durable medical equipment (DME)**: Medical equipment that has been prescribed by a health care provider that is either purchased or rented by a patient, to be used in the patient's home. Examples include hospital beds, walkers, canes, wheelchairs, oxygen, etc.

**Effect size**: The difference between the mean initial score (on an outcome instrument) and the mean follow-up score (on the same instrument) for a group of patients. Can be standardized by dividing the difference by the standard deviation of the initial scores.

**Environmental factors**: External factors, immediate or global, which affect the individual as he or she interacts with society; Can be physical, social, or attitudinal barriers, adaptations, or accommodations.

**Episode of (physical therapy) care**: All physical therapy services that are: 1) provided by a physical therapist, 2) provided in an unbroken sequence, and 3) related to the problem or related to a request from the patient/client, family, or other health care provider. The episode of care may include transfers between sites within or across settings or reclassification of the patient/client from one preferred practice pattern to another.

**Evaluation**: An assessment of the patient's condition based on data collected during the examination that is performed by the physical therapist. It includes consideration of the chronicity, severity, complexity, and extent of impairments, functional limitations, and disabilities.

**Evidence-based practice (EBP)**: Using the best evidence available along with clinical experience and patient values to make patient-care decisions.

**Examination**: A collection of tests and measurements, including questions to determine previous medical history, complaints, lifestyle, and physical therapy goals. The examination data is used to identify pertinent physical therapy problems, co-morbidities, rehabilitation potential, and to determine expected outcomes. It is also used to develop an plan of care that includes appropriate interventions, consultation with other health care providers, and patient education.

**Fiscal intermediary** (also known as **Intermediary**): A privately run insurance company that contracts with the government to pay bills for Medicare Part A and some Part B. Fiscal intermediaries are determined by geographic region and can be found at http://www.cms.hhs.gov/contacts/incardir.asp#4.

**Fraud**: Billing an insurance company, Medicare, or other third-party payer for services that were not provided, or billing for an item or service that has higher reimbursement than the service or item actually provided.

**Functional Independence Measure (FIM)**: A standardized, multidisciplinary evaluation tool often used to score the patient's performance in self-care, bowel and bladder management, transfers, gait and/or wheelchair mobility, communication, and cognition. Patients are scored 1 to 7 (1 equal to total assist and 7 equal to independent) according to the level of assist they require to complete the task.

**Functional limitation**: An abnormality, or limitation in an individual's ability to carry out a meaningful action, task, and/or activity, that is the result of a pathology and/or impairment(s).

**Functional outcome report (FOR)**: A format for documentation that focuses on the ability to perform meaningful functional activities rather than isolated musculoskeletal, neuromuscular, cardiopulmonary, or integumentary impairments.

**Goal**: The intended result of patient/client management. Goals indicate the change in body structure/ function, activity or participation limitation in functional and measurable time-limited goals.

**Health care clearinghouse**: An entity associated with a health care provider or third-party payer that provides services such as billing, database management, transcription, information technology, etc. The health care clearinghouse has access to patient information but is not involved in patient care.

**Health Insurance Portability and Accountability Act (HIPAA)**: A federal law enacted in 1996 that includes provisions for workers to maintain health insurance coverage when they change jobs, to safeguard privacy of a patient's confidential health information, and to combat health care fraud.

**History-taking**: Gathering of data—from the present and the past—related to why the patient is seeking physical therapy services. The data is collected through patient/family interviews, medical history review, and chart review.

**Home health care**: Skilled nursing or rehabilitative care provided in a patient's home. Home care services can be provided when a patient is declared "homebound."

**Homebound**: Status given to a patient when he is unable to leave his home, or when leaving requires significantly taxing efforts. Short, infrequent trips, such as medical appointments and religious services, are permitted when a patient has been declared "homebound."

**Impairment**: A deviation or loss in a body function or structure.

**Incident report**: A report filed in the event of an "incident" that could likely result in a lawsuit; Used to document errors and departures from normal procedures that result in adverse outcomes, procedural breakdowns, and catastrophic events. These reports are filed with the risk management department by the individual involved in the incident.

**Informed consent**: Consent to a treatment or service given by a patient after being informed of risks, benefits, alternatives, and consequences of no treatment at all.

**Inpatient Rehabilitation Facility (IRF)**: A hospital, or unit within a larger facility (ie, acute-care hospital), that provides intense rehabilitative services to patients. The majority of patients admitted to an IRF have been diagnosed with one of 13 qualifying medical conditions that have been established by Medicare. Examples are stroke, spinal cord injury, brain injury, amputation, hip fracture, burn, neurological disorder, and knee or hip replacement. More information and the list of qualifying diagnoses can be found at http://www.cms.hhs.gov/medlearn/matters/mmarticles/2004/MM3334.pdf.

**Interim note**: Part of the physical therapy documentation; Notes reflecting care provided after the initial examination and evaluation.

**Internal consistency**: A measurement of how "alike" individual items are in an instrument with multiple questions, or tasks to be performed.

**International Classification of Disease (ICD)**: A system of classifying patient illnesses and injuries by diagnosis. The tenth edition, ICD-10, is the most current version. The ninth edition, ICD-9, is still used commonly in the United States for insurance reimbursement purposes.

**International Classification of Functioning, Disabilities, and Health (ICF)**: A framework for evaluating and classifying consequences of disease endorsed by the World Health Organization.

**Inter-rater reliability**: The ability for multiple raters to obtain a consistent score on repeated attempts.

**Intervention**: Care provided to a patient or client by a physical therapist or physical therapist assistant; Includes coordination, communication, and documentation; patient/client-related instruction; and procedural interventions.

**Intraclass correlation coefficient (ICC)**: A reliability coefficient; A measurement of an instrument's reliability or repeatability.

**Intra-rater reliability**: The ability of one rater to obtain the same score on multiple attempts; Also known as **test-retest reliability**.

**Joint Commission on Accreditation of Health Care Organizations (JCAHO)**: An organization that accredits hospitals, ambulatory health care centers, home health agencies, and other health care organizations.

**Late entry**: A chart entry written after original documentation *and* other health care providers' documentation; Can also be written when enough time has elapsed so that the date of the late entry is different from the original documentation; The entry should be identified as a "late entry."

**Maintenance**: Services that can be provided by a non-licensed individual, including the patient himself, a family member, or a caregiver who has had some training from a skilled professional. Maintenance services are not reimbursed by Medicare or many other third-party payers.

**Malpractice**: A bad or unskillful act performed by a physician or other professional health care provider that injures or causes harm to a patient or client; Includes the failure of an individual or group to follow the accepted standards that have been set forth by their respective profession(s); Includes willful, negligent, and ignorant malpractice.

**Managed care**: A type of health care in which an insurance company (or third-party payer) maintains some control of costs and utilization of services and/or benefits.

**Measurement**: the numeral assigned to an object, event, or person or the class (category) to which an object, event, or person is assigned according to rules.

**Medical necessity**: As defined by Centers for Medicare & Medicaid Services, medical necessity is a procedure and/or intervention that is appropriate and needed for the diagnosis or treatment of a medical condition; is provided for the diagnosis, direct care, and treatment of a medical condition; meets the standards of good medical practice in the local area; and is not mainly for the convenience of the patient or health care provider.

**Medicare**: The federal health insurance program for individuals: 1) 65 years of age and older who are receiving or eligible for Social Security retirement benefits, 2) younger than 65 with certain disabilities who meet the Social Security Act's disability requirements, and 3) with end-stage renal disease. Medicare Part A typically pays for care provided by hospitals, skilled nursing facilities, and home health. Medicare Part B pays for physician services and outpatient-based care.

**Medicaid**: A joint federal and state program that helps with medical costs for individuals with low incomes and limited resources.

**Minimal clinical important difference (MCID)**: A value that represents an important, clinically significant change, which the patient also perceives as beneficial.

**Minimal detectable change (MDC)**: A value representing confidence of true change in a score rather than change due to error.

**Minimum Data Set (MDS)**: A standardized, multidisciplinary instrument used to collect data on patients in skilled nursing facilities. Data collected in the MDS is used to determine the amount Medicare will reimburse a facility for caring for a particular patient.

**Nagi framework**: A conceptual framework written by Saad Nagi linking components of pathology, impairment, functional limitation, and disability.

**Narrative note**: A documentation format in which pertinent information from the patient encounter is written as a paragraph.

**National Center for Medical Rehabilitation Research (NCMRR) disability classification scheme:** A conceptual framework for classifying pathophysiology, impairment, functional limitation, disability, and societal limitation set forth by the National Advisory Board on Medical Rehabilitation Research.

**Notice of Exclusion of Medicare Benefits (NEMB)**: A form or notice that a health care provider asks a Medicare beneficiary to sign when providing a service that is not covered by Medicare. In signing the NEMB, the Medicare beneficiary agrees to pay for the service not covered by Medicare (*see also* Advance Beneficiary Notice).

**Objective**: The O: portion of the SOAP note that includes measurable data or results of tests and measures, the patient's functional status, and interventions provided to a patient.

**Outcome**: The end result of patient/client management. Could also be the end result of an episode of care.

**Outcome and Assessment Information Set (OASIS)**: A standardized, multidisciplinary instrument used to collect information on patients receiving home health care. Medicare uses data on the OASIS to determine the amount of payment a home health agency will receive for providing care to a patient.

**Participation**: Involvement in life situations and performance of social skills, such as in work or community involvement.

**Participation restrictions**: Problems an individual faces while involved in life situations.

**Pathology**: The interference with the body's normal processes and simultaneous body efforts to heal itself, or regain a normal state. Often known as the actual disease or medical diagnosis.

**Patient/Client Management Model**: A model outlined and depicted in *The Guide to Physical Therapist Practice* describing physical therapist management of a patient or client; Includes a description of examination, evaluation, diagnosis, prognosis (including the plan of care), and interventions.

**Performance**: Measured on the ICF evaluation scheme; Includes the extent of the individual's participation restrictions, or actual performance in his or her current environment. It is scored according to how much difficulty the individual experiences in life situations and performance of social skills, such as in work or community involvement, assuming the person wants to participate.

**Personal factors**: Individual characteristics, ie, age, race, gender, co-morbidities, etc.

**Plan**: The P: portion of a SOAP note; Indicates communication/collaboration, patient/client-related education and procedural interventions that are a part of the physical therapy plan of care; includes the clinician's intentions for future interventions.

**Plan of care**: A plan describing which interventions a patient will receive during the episode of care; Includes the amount, frequency, and duration of services to be provided, and may also include the expected final outcome(s).

**Practice act**: A law, typically enacted by a state legislature, which governs the practice of a profession. All 50 states have practice acts that provide for licensure of physical therapists.

**Premium**: A payment made to an insurance company to cover an individual under an insurance plan. Premiums are typically paid monthly. Many employers pay a portion of an employee's monthly premium as a benefit of employment. The insurance company pools the premiums received for a large group of individuals to pay the health care costs of those in the group.

**Primary care provider (PCP)**: A physician responsible for a patient's point-of-entry into the health care system. Some insurance companies require the PCP to be the patient's family physician. It can also be a general practitioner, internal medicine specialist, or in some cases an obstetrician/gynecologist.

**Problem list**: A list of impairments and/or functional limitations that will be addressed during an episode of care. May also include co-morbidities, complexities, or complicating factors.

**Problem-oriented medical record (POMR)**: A documentation format organized according to the patient's problems; Includes a patient-problem list that serves as a "table of contents" for the remainder of the medical record; Subsequent entries include status and treatment for individual problems.

**Prognosis**: Includes anticipated goals, the expected outcome(s), and may also include the ultimate plan for discharge; Also includes the patient's potential for achieving his or her goals.

**Progress Report/Note**: A special type of interim note that provides evidence for ongoing medical necessity of treatment; Includes subjective and objective data, an assessment of patient progress including his or her status toward existing goals; Also includes changes to the existing goals or plan of care, as well as justification for these changes.

**Prospective Payment System (PPS)**: Medicare reimbursement provided to facilities (ie, hospitals and skilled nursing facilities) that is predetermined, or fixed, based on the patient's diagnosis and/or complexity.

**Protected health information (PHI)**: Individually identifiable information referring to an individual's medical history; previous, current, and future medical care; and billing and/or payment information, also known as **individually identifiable health information**. Also includes information that could potentially allow identification of the individual, eg, address, telephone and fax number, birth date, admission and discharge dates, voice recordings.

**Provider**: An individual (such as a physical therapist or physician) or an organization (such as a hospital) that provides health care to patients.

**Re-examination/Re-evaluation:** A separately payable service performed by a physical therapist when the assessment indicates a significant improvement, decline, or change in condition or functional status that was not anticipated; Formal, thorough, complete records of the patient's status, including tests and measures from the initial encounter, any additional tests and measures, record of new developments or problems the patient may be having; Includes specific progress (or lack thereof) toward goals stated on the plan of care; Can also occur within a required time frame dictated by law, a payer, or facility policy.

**Regulation**: A rule established by a governmental agency, which has been granted such authority by Congress or a state legislature.

**Reimbursement**: Payment made to a health care provider from an insurance company, or other third-party payer after being billed for a service provided to a patient.

**Reliability**: The repeatability, or consistency, with which an instrument or rater is able to measure a variable.

**Responsiveness**: An instrument's sensitivity to change.

**Resource Utilization Group (RUG)**: Refers to the classification system used by Medicare to determine payment for care in skilled nursing facilities. Each patient in this setting is classified into one of 53 different RUG categories based on the types and intensity of services required to care for the patient. The skilled nursing facility is paid a daily rate to care for the patient; the daily rate is adjusted to account for the patient's RUG category.

**Review of Systems (ROS)**: *See* **Systems review.**

**Secondary insurance**: Additional or supplemental insurance carried by a patient. The secondary will typically cover additional costs not covered by the individual's primary insurance.

**Skilled care:** A type of health care given when a patient needs management, observation, or evaluation by trained nurses or rehabilitation staff; also includes care that requires the unique judgment and/or skill of a trained individual for both safety and effectiveness.

**Skilled Nursing Facility (SNF)**: A free-standing facility (or facility within a hospital, nursing home, or rehabilitation center) that provides skilled medical, nursing, or rehabilitative services to patients. Examples of skilled services include intravenous injections, oxygen, feeding tubes, wound care, and rehabilitation (http://www.cms.hhs.gov/manuals/cmstoc.asp).

**SOAP note**: A documentation format where information is arranged according to the headings S:, O:, A:, and P:, or subjective, objective, assessment, and plan, respectively.

**Standard error of the measurement (SEM)**: Quantification of the reliability, given in the same measurement units as the original measurement.

**Standardized response mean (SRM)**: A measure of an instrument's responsiveness or sensitivity to change; Calculated by taking the difference between the mean of the initial score (on an outcome instrument) and the mean follow-up score (on the same instrument) and

then dividing by the standard deviation of the change scores.

**State practice act**: A state's regulation of licensed professionals. Usually defines the educational requirements, licensure requirements, scope of practice, acceptable service delivery, and continuing education requirements.

**Subjective**: The S: portion of the SOAP note; Information regarding the patient's status/condition provided by the patient, a family member, or a caregiver; Includes the history-taking portion of the examination.

**Systems review:** Part of the data collection procedures during a physical therapy examination; Includes a gross review of body systems and measuring vital signs; Used to guide decision-making as to what tests and measures should be performed during the remainder of the examination.

**Test**: A set of procedures that is used to obtain measurements (data); The procedures may require the use of instruments.

**Tests and Measures:** Specific standardized methods and techniques used to gather data about the patient/client after the history and systems review have been performed.

**Test-retest reliability**: *See* **intra-rater reliability**.

**Third-party payer**: The insurance company or other entity that pays for medical services provided to a patient. The patient and the health care provider are considered the primary parties.

**Treatment note**: *See* **interim note**.

**Validity**: The degree that an instrument or rater measures the variable that it (or he) intends to measure.

**World Health Organization (WHO)**: The directing and coordinating authority for health within the United Nations system. It is responsible for providing leadership on global health matters, shaping the health research agenda, setting norms and standards, articulating evidence-based policy options, providing technical support to countries, and monitoring and assessing health trends (http://www.who.int/about/en/).

# Index

# WAIT
## ...There's More!

SLACK Incorporated's Health Care Books and Journals offers a wide selection of products in the field of Physical Therapy. We are dedicated to providing important works that educate, inform and improve the knowledge of our customers. Don't miss out on our other informative titles that will enhance your collection.

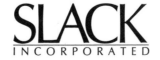